HALO FOUND

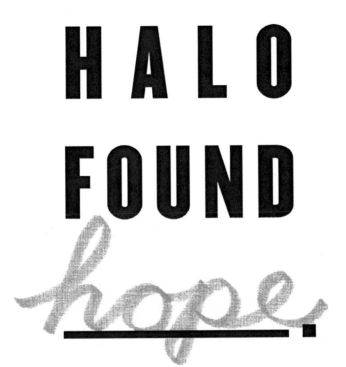

hope

A MEMOIR

HELO MATZELLE

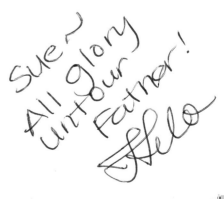

First published by Dog Ear Publishing
4010 W. 86th Street, Ste H
Indianapolis, IN 46268
www.dogearpublishing.net

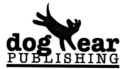

ISBN: 978-1-4575-3133-0

Library of Congress Control Number: has been applied for

This book is printed on acid-free paper.

Printed in the United States of America

CONTENTS

This book is dedicated to

The One

In whom true hope is found.

Introduction

Hi, my first name is Helouise, but I've gone by the nickname Helo, pronounced "Halo" my entire life. When people see or hear my name for the first time they often ask me, "How is your name spelled and pronounced?" Then I explain, "It's spelled with an 'e' but pronounced with an 'a'—Halo, like an angel has a halo on its head." Then I often receive a comment like, "You must be an angel"—to which I softly respond, "No, I am not." I've had mixed feelings about this description (growing up with a name that no one can pronounce isn't exactly easy), but it has served as a great icebreaker when I meet people.

I was named after my grandmother, Helouise, on my dad's side. People frequently ask me what my nationality is. My dad is part black, Chinese, and Portuguese, and my mom is German and Swedish. It's made forms that ask for racial background a little annoying, since I get tired of checking boxes, and it's led to me wanting to create a box just labeled "human." However, my husband finds it hilarious to be married to a woman with such a colorful background, and likes to call me his "Heinz 57 ®" beauty.

My father is from Suriname, a former Dutch colony, and my mother is from Germany. They met in the Netherlands while my dad was studying to become a physicist. On October 19, 1964, in the city of Delft, I came into this world with a full head of hair that never stopped growing. In the hospital, shocked by my impressive locks, the nurses chose to christen me as a lost member of The Beatles. My family had nicknames for me, too. They sometimes said, "Hello, Weasel" in place of Helouise. My mom, in her fun German accent, called me Veasie. My family sang a song to me in the classic tune of "Hello Dolly."[1] The words went like this: "Oh hello, Weasel, oh hello, Weasel, it's so nice to have a sister [or daughter] just like you." I loved their choice of melody, but didn't like to be associated with weasels...or bugs.

1

Three months after my birth, my parents decided to immigrate from the Netherlands to the United States, in order to pursue better opportunities for the little family they had started. Boarding a ship, they traveled across the Atlantic Ocean with only three hundred guilders (about two hundred dollars) to their name. I slept in a makeshift crib: a suitcase with the lid tied to the bed. Of course, my mom didn't sleep well, terrified that the lid would close on her baby daughter during the night.

My dad took on a postdoctoral fellowship at Northwestern University in Evanston, Illinois. It was the mid-1960's, and my parents experienced discrimination as a result of their mixed marriage, which was illegal in eighteen states at the time. But my mom and dad loved each other, and they knew I needed a little brother. On August 25, 1966, my brother, Henk, was born in Chicago.

During his physics career, my dad declined a position at the Scandia National Laboratories due to its association with weapons research. He refused the offer because during World War II, my mom had spent the early years of her childhood in a bunker during bombing raids. The alarms had sounded and she had hid underground for safety. This terror scarred my mom for life.

At the end of 1966, my family moved to Seattle, Washington, where my dad joined the faculty at the University of Washington to teach physics. After several years, my family moved to Florida, where my dad attended the PhD-to-MD program at the University of Miami to become a medical doctor and specialize in the field of rehabilitation medicine. My mom worked hard as a secretary to put my dad through medical school, and to raise me and my brother with much love. While in rehabilitation practice, my dad worked as a hospice MD to help patients who were suffering from terminal illnesses, and to assist the family members standing by their sides.

My brother and I had fun growing up. Games were always simple. When we lived in Miami, we threw coconuts from the third floor of our apartment onto the concrete sidewalks to crack open the shells. Of course, it was never really that simple. First we had to find the coconuts, and if there wasn't one on the ground, we had to shake it down from the tree. We must have looked like monkeys, two kids shaking a tree violently and waiting for something to fall off. Then, if we were lucky, a brown, ripe coconut would fall; we could husk it, poke holes into it with a screwdriver, and get at the milk. We would drink it and enjoy the beverage. However, we still had to try to crack it open. But, of course, coconuts are hard. So, in order to get at the sweet, white coconut meat, my brother would carry the coconut up three stories to the roof, while I kept watch below to make sure no heads were injured as the coconut catapulted down from above. Finally, we'd break out the spoons and eat our snack, after having expended far more calories to get it than we gained in eating it.

After my dad finished medical school, our family moved back to Seattle. My brother and I enjoyed our teenage years together and got along well. We missed each other when I left for college, even though I lived close by.

I attended the University of Washington and met my future husband there. The first time I met him, I thought he was handsome. The second time I met him, I was impressed he remembered my name. The third time, I thought he was cute and funny, but way too playful and totally not my type. I was wrong about that. Rich grew to love me because of who I was inside, and I fell in love with him, too. Rich is patient, kind, fun, caring, and adorable. I've been so blessed.

We got married on April 22, 1989, and moved to Utah, living away from our parents and siblings for seven years. Rich continued his career right out of college with IBM. After college graduation, I worked three, part-time jobs for several months while interviewing for full-time work. I finally landed my first "real job" working for Bristol-Meyers Squibb, a worldwide pharmaceutical company marketing prescription medications to doctors and their staff.

I felt accomplished in my career pursuits. When we had our first child, Lauren, I became a stay-at-home mom. It was rewarding and intense. All of a sudden, I had a new appreciation for how much work it was to be a mom—either one who worked outside of the home or stayed home. Rich and I wanted to have more children, but we experienced the significant challenge of conceiving and then losing them. It brought us closer. Later, God blessed us with two additional amazing children.

I was a busy and faithful wife, devoted mom, caring daughter, loving sister, and dedicated friend. I loved God, family, and friends tenaciously. I cherished the wonderful things in my life and didn't take any of it for granted, or so I thought. Life was busyness, blessings, and excitement. I had a beautiful home, a great husband, incredible children, and a cute dog named Grace.

Then one day, everything changed; my life came to a complete stand-still. Facing potential death early in life is scary. Learning that you have a brain tumor that needs immediate surgery changes your perspective quickly. Earthly obligations were abruptly set aside. I was pushed to a place that I had never been to before—brought to a complete and terrifying halt. And then the challenge of having to learn just about everything, that the brain controls, over again, consumed me. My family and I were trans-formed and grew closer to each other. We gained a greater understanding of who God is, and I fell in love with Him more than I ever imagined pos-sible.

It was as if God said to me, "Helo, I did not pull you through this incredible journey without a purpose. There's a story I want you to share. The affliction was hard, and the miracle that unfolded was magnificent and humbling. It showed you how much I love you, and each and every indi-vidual whom I created."

I never thought that I would write a book. This one started out as a diary about a nightmare that I'd never dreamed of experiencing. After a long day, it was hard for me to fall asleep. My mind raced. I got up and went down to the home office to type out my thoughts, and ended up back in bed too late. After weeks of this, my husband placed a notepad on the nightstand by the bed so I wouldn't have to go downstairs anymore.

Night after night, thoughts filled my mind and then the notepads on my nightstand. I had hopes that if I put the thoughts on paper, my mind would stop racing; I'd become still and fall asleep. This didn't work. I'd pick up the pad again at one or two a.m. I didn't want to wake my husband, so I scribbled in the dark. I thought that I was being clever by not turning on the light, but Rich heard the pen scratching on the pad and the pages turning. He's a patient man, so after about an hour, he'd tell me it was time to stop and go to sleep. Then morning came and it was hard to read my handwriting. I had written notes over other notes. Writing in the dark is messy.

"And God said, 'Let there be light,' and there was light."[2] God created light for a reason. I continued to write in the dark for months on end, sometimes even waking up in the middle of the night. I couldn't fall back asleep until my thoughts were scribbled down. Writing during the day was better, and much was accomplished. God and I were having a great time together, but at times, I wondered why I was writing a story. Writing takes a lot of brain power. My brain was traumatized, so writing was emotionally and intellectually exhausting. Sometimes writing was cathartic. Other times, it made me weary.

One day, I went into Costco to get gas. Stevy, a contagiously joyful man, approached me to offer help and then pointed out an eagle in the sky. I exclaimed, "Wow, God made that eagle, and it's beautiful!"

Stevy mentioned that no other customer had made a comment like that about the eagle that he pointed out often. I shared my story with him and mentioned that I'd considered writing a book but that it was hard for me. He told me, "Sister, you have a story to share!" Then I remembered, "…but those who hope in the Lord will renew their strength. They will soar on wings like eagles; they will run and not grow weary, they will walk, and not be faint."[3]

Time is precious. Thank you for carving out moments of your busy day to read this. May you be encouraged to find hope.

Chapter One

BROUGHT TO A HALT

...I will lead them in paths they have not known. I will make darkness light before them, and crooked places straight.

— Isaiah 42:16 NKJV —

On October 19, 2010 I turned forty-six. I got to celebrate being a year older with my family. My husband held my hand as we walked behind our three children. They were goofing off, laughing, and joking around with each other. It delighted us. Lauren was in her last year of college, our son Jordan had just started high school, and Austin was in junior high. The five of us had gone to an open-air Mexican restaurant on the water. I opened a small basket filled with thoughtful birthday gifts as we laughed and my family told funny stories about me.

After leaving the restaurant we walked along the waterfront. Being together was the best birthday gift of all. I had it really good: a strong faith in God, a great husband, beautiful kids, a comfortable home, and good health. Or so I thought.

Then in the months that followed, I began to experience odd sensations. I would hear clear voices in my head at random. I heard voices talking—characters interacting. Puzzled, I would stop whatever I was doing, close my eyes, and try to figure out what movie clip they were from. Then the voices suddenly stopped and I experienced a brief metallic taste in my mouth. The taste quickly vanished and I felt like I was going to faint, but I didn't, so I went on with my day. This happened about a dozen times over a two month period; the majority of these symptoms took place while I was in a building that was painted often. I attributed my peculiar sensations to the intensity of the paint vapors.

The symptoms were so brief and so odd that I thought no one would believe me even if I described them. When I shared them with my husband, Rich, he reminded me that he was not a doctor. I told my dad, now a retired physician, about the strange symptoms, and he attributed them to stress. So, I tried to ignore them. I was such a busy wife and mom that my dad's reasoning made sense. Two years later, I learned from my neurosurgeon that these symptoms were the result of auditory hallucination seizures.

Additionally, I had ringing in both ears for more than a year, which was annoying, but tolerable. I learned later that this actually had nothing to do with my tumor, but it was for this symptom that I went to see a doctor. The noise in my right ear got so loud at night that I could not sleep. Perhaps I was paying way too much attention to the noise.

In January of 2011, I scheduled an appointment to get my ears checked. I had lost fifty percent of the hearing in my right ear, which was masked by the constant ringing. Dr. Calvin Knapp, an ear, nose, and throat (ENT) physician, whom I had known for years, ordered an MRI with a dye-contrast study on my ear as a precautionary first step to solving my hearing loss and to rule out a benign tumor in my ear. If this was discovered, outpatient surgery would restore my hearing.

It was a Friday afternoon, and I asked Dr. Knapp if I could get the results that day. I did not want to worry about it over the weekend. After the MRI, I sat in the busy waiting room thinking, "*I've got multiple errands to run, tasks to complete, dinner guests coming over, my son's basketball game to attend, church on Sunday, date night with my husband, and school projects to help with.*" I was planning for the days ahead—and the "to-do" list went on.

I knew something was up when Dr. Knapp's nurse, Tara, escorted me back to the examination room. Her usually cheerful face dimmed. I did not have to wait for the doctor this time; he was waiting for me, and he had brought in backup. Dr. Knapp looked calm, but concerned. Tara left me there, with the doctors, but I was confused. What was the second doctor for?

Fear began to sink in.

I asked Dr. Knapp, "This isn't something simple, is it?"

He locked eyes with me, and then with a concerned look said, "No, Helo, it isn't."

I thought, "*What in the world is this about?*" My heart started to race.

In a compassionate and gentle way, he continued, "Helo, this has absolutely nothing to do with your hearing loss. You have a brain tumor the size of a golf ball sitting over the carotid (main) artery in your brain."

Silence.

I was in a state of complete shock—and confused.

Startled, I shook my head, looked right at him, bent back and forth with my arms crossed, and stuttered, "What did you just say?"

Dr. Knapp calmly repeated, "Helo, you have a brain tumor."

Puzzled, I stared at him, "Really?"

Stillness.

Softly he said, "Yes."

I thought to myself, "*A few hours ago, I was just fine. I was a devoted wife, busy mom, who led a healthy and active life. I had ringing in both ears. Lots of people have that. Annoying? Yes! Life threatening? No! I was planning my weekend. Now, I had a brain tumor in my head. Someone please tell me this isn't happening—this does not feel real.*"

"Please get my dad on the phone so that he can listen in on our conversation."

Dr. Knapp grabbed the phone and asked me for my dad's number. He dialed and handed it to me. I was shaking so much that I could hardly hold onto the phone. I knew that my dad could explain later whatever was happening. I also needed the comfort of him listening in.

I prayed quietly to my Heavenly Father, "*Please shelter my mind and heart.*" Worried on the inside, shaking on the outside, I needed His assurance. God whispered to me, "Be still, and know that I am God."[1] It was time for me to believe that God would walk alongside me. With Him, I could live through and endure anything, even though I had no idea what was about to happen.

My dad picked up the line.

"Dad, it's me. I'm at Dr. Knapp's office in an examination room with him and another doctor. I need you to talk to them."

"Are you okay?"

"No."

"What's going on, Helo?"

After a long and awkward pause, I quietly said, "Dad, I have a brain tumor."

"What?"

"I have a brain tumor. I need Dr. Knapp to explain what's going on." I could hardly talk anymore. Trembling, I handed over the phone, and it was placed on speaker.

"Dr. Knapp, are you sure?"

"Yes, Henk."

Then the other doctor added, "She needs to go in for surgery as soon as possible."

My dad insisted, "I need details."

And then the two doctors in the room talked with my dad for awhile. I don't remember what they discussed. It sounded like they were using a lot of big words that I did not understand.

I wanted to turn back the hands of time and erase the incidental diagnosis. I knew that God had the power to do so, but He also had the power to allow this for a reason that I could not yet understand. My eyes welled up with tears. Still in shock, I began to shake uncontrollably. My mind was racing, and I began to panic.

"Why this, God?"

The other doctor excused himself, got up from his chair, left the room, and closed the door behind him.

Dr. Knapp asked, "How long will it take your parents to get here?"

"About half an hour."

"Would you like me to call your husband?"

"No, I'll do that," I replied.

"Helo, I've arranged for you to see the best neurosurgeon on Monday afternoon. If my wife had to have surgery on her brain, he's the one I would send her to. You are going to be in excellent hands."

"Thanks," I whispered.

This was not easy for Dr. Knapp, either. "Helo, you can wait in this exam room if you want to."

"I'd rather go sit outside."

He picked up my coat, helped me put it on, opened the door, and I left the room. I walked in a daze down the hallway, out the door, into the parking lot, and sat on a curb in the rain. Sobbing.

I never imagined that something like this could ever happen to me.

The day I was diagnosed with a brain tumor brought me to a terrifying halt. It was as if God had said to me, "My cherished and beloved child, it is time for you to be completely still. The gift I have given you, of being a wife, is at a standstill. Motherly duties are on complete hold. Everyday tasks of family life that you hold so important do not matter as much as you think. Life here on earth is temporary, my dear. You are here to be molded, and one day you will meet Me and my Son. Rely and focus on Me. *Trust Me.* I made you, will forever love you, and I will never leave you alone." It was time for me to recognize that not everything we "plan" will happen the way we assume it will. God is in control—we are not.

I asked Jesus to cradle me and shower me with love. I called my husband, Rich. He was busy at work but immediately agreed to meet me at home; he was shocked by the inconceivable news as well. Overcome with fear and worry, I could not get behind the wheel to drive home; I was sobbing too much. This moment in time felt surreal. *It could not be happening.*

My dad and mom came to pick me up at the doctor's office. Half an hour passed by while I waited, and as they drove into the parking lot, I wept again. We locked eyes. My mom privately thought that I was shaking like a little bird, as I sat on that curb in the rain. They quietly got out of their car without even parking in a spot or closing the car doors behind them; they held onto me, and none of us wanted to let the others go. Any discord, that I had ever had with them in my past, completely vanished as I thought of the many reasons that I loved them. Dad told me, "Everything will be all right." What father would want to say anything different to his adored child?

I silently cried out to my Heavenly Father, *"Your beloved needs you now. Don't let go of me. Please take this and give me strength."* I desperately needed Him to prepare me for what lay ahead. I never thought I would walk a road like this one. Dad drove me home in my car, and my mom drove home in Dad's car. I still don't know how she handled driving alone after hearing my terrifying news.

As my parents walked with me into the house, I was paralyzed by the thought that this might be the last time I would come home. I knew that I was going to see an exceptional surgeon, but... Within moments my husband was home. We were both shaken, but he was stronger than I was. He took my hand, held on tightly, and walked me upstairs to our room. Tears ran down my face as I looked at him and cried out, "Why?—Tell me this isn't really happening." He held me tenderly. The love of my life cradled me in his arms and did not let go.

Rich said, "I love you, Helo. Everything will be okay.

Shock fertilizes fear. Fear shatters hope. But hope found moves faith to blossom again. Faith restored allows peace and courage to take hold.

— Helo

We prayed and asked God to help us both; now we would not walk alone. We decided to hold off telling our children about my condition, until after we learned more. Monday was to be my appointment with a neurosurgeon. It was so hard for me to fully enjoy the weekend with my family. My kids had no idea why I hugged them so many times, and told them over and over again, "I love you." I watched them play board and card games, run around the house, make messes, shoot hoops with my husband, do homework, gobble up dinner, and play with our dog Grace. Every time my kids made me laugh, I wanted to cry at the thought that this *might* be the last time I'd see them so happy. There was no forgetting what was going on, and while I knew that telling my children would only lead to questions we couldn't answer, it hurt to know that soon we would have to share terrible news…whatever that terrible news was.

Monday arrived, and we saw Dr. James Raisis, a renowned neurosurgeon in Seattle. He's an excellent physician who has stated that it is a privilege to be able to operate on a patient's brain. Dr. Raisis enjoys getting to know both the patient and the patient's family. He reviewed my MRI results and described the danger of the brain tumor lying over the carotid artery, which is the main artery to and from the brain. Without blood flow, the brain would "starve" and could die. There was also the threat of a grand mal seizure. I started an anti-seizure medication immediately and plans were made to enter the hospital the following Monday.

The next step was to tell our kids. *It broke our hearts.*

We all sat around the kitchen table. Typically we sat there to share a meal, play games, tell stories, and laugh.

This time was different.

I sat there feeling numb, so Rich quietly started the conversation.

"Kids, Mom and I have something difficult to tell you."

Their smiles faded.

"Mom has a brain tumor. Today we met with a specialist, and he told us that she needs to have it removed as soon as possible. I'm taking her to the hospital next Monday."

They looked at us in disbelief.

Silence.

Rich took a deep breath, and then did his best to reassure our kids.

"Mom is going to be okay. She is under the care of a phenomenal neurosurgeon, Dr. Raisis, and his medical team. She will be in the hospital for only six days. When she comes home, we'll give her lots of TLC. She'll need to take it easy for about two weeks."

Rich has a way of remaining strong and calm. Our kids accepted the news, we prayed, and they told me how much they loved me. I held it together, gave them each a hug, repeated, "I love you too," and told them that I was going to be "okay."

Then I thought, *"Be brave, Helo."*

I reminded myself that in twenty-nine years of practice, my neurosurgeon only had one other patient stay in the hospital for more than a week. I would be in good hands. Ultimately, I was in God's hands. But on the inside, I felt paralyzed by the uncertainty of returning home again. I didn't want to show my kids how scared I was, so I hurried up to my room, sat on the floor, and sobbed. I felt frail and fearful. Fear is poison that either discourages hope or pushes us to seek it. I needed hope.

Chapter Two

PUMMELED BY FEAR

*Worry does not empty tomorrow of its sorrow,
it empties today of its strength.*

— Corrie ten Boom —

Satan delights in pulling down those who seek hope. Worry makes us vulnerable to the enemy, who wants us to focus upon defeat as a battle begins. *My diagnosis turned my world upside down.* I could choose to seek hope or to give up. If I gave up, Satan would nourish fearful thoughts. He wanted me to panic, cry out in angry desperation, and wonder where God was in all of this. I admit that I did cry out and panic, yielding to fear. I confess I had moments when I allowed Satan in as I doubted God. There were times I convinced myself that I had totally failed my Heavenly Father by not trusting Him, and became discouraged. In those moments I'd turn and "scream" at Satan to get away from me, and remind myself, *"Fear entices the enemy; faith brings us closer to God."*

During those battles, it was as if God said, "Helo, listen to me. Do you trust me?"

I put my trust in Him, and found safety. "I will say of the Lord, He is my refuge and my fortress; my God; in Him I will trust."[1]

I chose to allow God to take the best and worst of me, because He is the One to trust. I won't write much about Satan in this book because he doesn't deserve our time, unless we are telling him to back off—even then he doesn't deserve our attention, he just wants it. Satan takes our weak points and delights in embellishing them.

Give your attention to God instead. He takes our weaknesses, when we relinquish them to Him, then graces us with courage, peace, and endurance—and makes us stronger. He imparts hope to the hopeless, rest to the restless, courage to the discouraged. As C. S. Lewis once wrote, "There is no neutral ground in the universe: every square inch, every split second, is claimed by God and counterclaimed by Satan." But the good news is—God always overpowers the enemy.

God Is Stronger Than the Enemy Because...

Hope withstands the force of fear.
Faith and trust are stronger than doubt.
Peace covers anger.
Love replaces hate.
God's promises wipe out lies and deception.
Prayers erase confusion.
Compassion defies insensitivity.
Endurance replaces quitting.
Joy outlives pain.
Light dispels darkness.
Beauty redeems ashes.
The promise of Heaven makes the fear of death disappear.
Battles given to God are won.
The promise that hope can be found gives us the courage
to go on.

— Helo

The discovery of my brain tumor was the first of many miracles that I experienced. The purpose of the MRI ordered by my ENT was to evaluate my ear in order to rule out a treatable concern. When an MRI is done for an ear problem, the brain is coincidentally viewed at the same time because of its proximity to the ear. Receiving confirmation that my hearing loss was due to a treatable concern would have been so much easier to deal with. But had the brain tumor been discovered much later, it could have strangled the carotid artery, threatening my life. To complicate matters, I could have a grand mal seizure at any time, and potentially die.

Prior to surgery, Dr. Raisis spent over twenty hours focusing on my case. He didn't know whether the tumor could be entirely removed because it was precariously wrapping itself around the carotid and potentially invading the sinus cavity. *It was located in a very dangerous place.* Later, there would be medical discussion about having the carotid grafted, but this procedure could be life-threatening in and of itself. There was also the concern that even if I came out of surgery, I could become vegetative. Even so, God granted me and my family the courage to go on. He is a mighty God, full of mercy, fortitude, and grace. "So do not fear, for I am with you; do not be dismayed, for I am your God. I will strengthen you and help you; I will uphold you with my righteous right hand."[2]

Now nothing on earth mattered to me except my family and close friends. What kind of home I lived in, the car I drove, and my worldly achievements in life had no significance. I reflected on the legacy I would leave behind if I died, *"What kind of wife and mom was I? Had I been the daughter, sister, and friend that God would be proud of?"* Though I had an incredibly loving family surrounding me, I felt alone. Confusion and dreaded apprehension smothered me.

I was scared to death of dying—not because I wasn't sure where I would go, I knew that Heaven was waiting for me—I was frightened for the family that I might leave behind, and overwhelmed with all that we would miss out on if I died: Every birthday, Christmas, Easter, graduation, wedding, and grandchild. Days of growing old—that wouldn't happen.

"Who will be the wife, mom, daughter, and sister to those that I love? Who will love my husband and tell him what a wonderful man he is, and encourage him? Who will hug my children and love them like I do?" These excruciating questions gave way to smaller concerns: *"Who will make dinner? Help them with school? Clean the house? Run errands? Manage the household? Care for the roses?"* And then I leapt into preparation mode—or rather, preoccupation mode. I was doing my best to deal with what lay ahead, but self-reliance did not help.

In my busyness as a wife, mom, and friend, I sometimes thought that I was too busy to read my Bible, or take precious time to slow down and pray. Some days were filled with spending time with Him, but on other days, I set Him aside and vowed, "God, I promise that I will spend quality and quantity time with you tomorrow. I'm sorry; I just cannot fit it in today." Then tomorrow came, the pattern repeated, and my promise was broken.

As I waited to be admitted for surgery, I finally understood that it is sweeter not to allow busyness to consume my day. I had gone to church all my life, called myself a Christian, and thought that my relationship with God was as good as it could be. Now, that was changing. Knowing my Maker was more than just going to church, and labeling myself as someone with faith. I was falling in love with Him all over again. Hope was found, and encouragement took hold of "today." I learned to carve out time for God, making Him my first priority. Doing so made my "todays" beautiful even while I faced brain tumor removal. I learned to trust Him even more, and He revealed time and time again, how much He loves me. Overwhelming loneliness lessened, minute by minute at times.

Still, I kept busy to suppress my lingering distress. I diligently planned ahead to organize the home, make meals in advance, and run errands. Michael, my friend and hairdresser for over a decade, from Gene Juarez Hair Salon, graciously offered to visit my home to cut and style my hair two days before I went in for hospital admission. He set up a makeshift salon in my master bathroom upstairs, took gentle care of me, styled my hair, and made me feel pretty. We both knew that in a few days, the left side of my head would be shaved entirely bald, but I needed a normal moment because what I was facing felt surreal. My hair was cut and styled now, because many weeks would pass before I could visit the salon again. Michael has a tender way of listening. I cried, but that was okay. Being nervous about the upcoming surgery, I didn't want to go to the hair salon and be around other clients and hairdressers. After recovery, I would visit the salon again.

The day before surgery, I went shopping at Nordstrom with my parents to get comfortable pajamas for when I came home. All three of us walked through the store in a fog, trying to occupy our minds with practical tasks. But as soon as the dressing room door closed behind me, I sank to the chair, shaking and sobbing. All I could think was, *"Why am I trying these on? I may never get to wear them."* I tried them on anyway. They fit. I pulled myself together—I didn't want my parents to see me like this—and left the dressing room, pajamas in hand.

As I stood at the counter, I wondered if I should buy a present for each one of my kids. But a present wasn't what we all needed. I wanted to drop the pajamas right then and there, run home to my family, and spend the last moments before surgery with the people I love most.

The salespeople at Nordstrom are enthusiastic, helpful, and kind, but I couldn't bring myself to talk to anyone in the store except my parents. The woman at the counter told me to, "Have a nice evening." I couldn't bring myself to tell her what kind of evening I was actually going to have.

As we walked out of the store, I asked my father about the upcoming surgery. I was scared and I was scared enough to let him see. My father is an optimistic man. But in this moment I didn't want his optimism, I wanted reality. He told me it was probably a benign meningioma and that I would be "okay." I got mad. I didn't want fake reassurances.

"Dad, if you are trying to placate me, it is not going to work. If you think for even a moment that I might not make it, I want to write letters to Rich and the kids and videotape messages for future milestones in their lives."

"Helo, if I thought for even a second that you wouldn't make it, I'd go home with you right now and help you videotape any message you want."

I thought to myself, *"I would still like to write letters to the kids in case I die. Maybe I should, and then pray that the kids won't have to read them until I am eighty."*

Dad, why is this happening?"

"I don't know, Helo. I wish it wasn't. I love you."

"I love you, too."

At that moment I knew how much my parents loved me, but it wasn't enough. Only God could love me the amount that I needed. I missed my kids and wanted to hurry home. Time felt like it was being whisked away. I had once enjoyed shopping, but it was hard this night. My mom held one of my hands, and my dad the other, as we left. If I got through the surgery and recovery, I'd come back.

My husband was at work, finalizing projects, preparing to take time off. I got home and hugged my children. My husband's and children's love did not erase my terrifying thoughts; rather, their love fueled my fear. As they showed compassion for me, I was hit with the stark reality again that I could potentially be leaving them for good. I might not be here for graduations, weddings, and grandchildren. *This was heartbreaking.* My family did their best to show me how much they loved me, but even their transparent affection did not erase moments of my feeling isolated. So I pulled God into my solitary place of suffering and was no longer alone.

I switched back and forth from "staying busy" to feeling overwhelmed by fear. *"Flash-forward, Helo, in about ten days, you'll be back home. Focus on the future instead of the trouble that you are about to face."* I cleaned the house while sobbing. Enough. Time to be still. Being "still" was hard, because time felt like it was evaporating. It is impossible to freeze, rewind, or fast-forward time and I was facing a countdown. Anxiety can be mean—so I asked God to take off my chains of trepidation. Weeping, I wanted to know, *"Where are you taking me with all of this?"* I fell to my knees and whispered, "I feel alone. I am too young to die and love my family too much to leave them. God, I still have so much to do. I am scared to leave those I love, even though I know that if I do, I will be with You in Heaven. Jesus, please continually comfort them and stay by their sides if I leave. And never let any of us go."

After wailing to the point that there were no more tears to shed, I immersed myself in the moment—anchored in constant prayer. I was doing my best to focus on one day at a time, with God's steadfast help. This was completely new to me. My relationship with Jesus intensified to the point that I asked Him to walk by my side every second. I cried out to God, "Please make something beautiful out of this."

God reminded me again, "Be still and know that I am God."[3] He also declared, "Have I not commanded you? Be strong and courageous. Do not be terrified; do not be discouraged, for the Lord your God will be with you wherever you go."[4]

It was time for me to trust Him.

I finally learned that we cannot find peace or comfort by planning excessively or trying to control our future, but that is what I did in an attempt to quench my fear. I was terrified by my brain tumor diagnosis. That was completely normal. Fear contorts and destroys the pursuit of hope, but God is not intimidated by the enemy. Eventually, I chose to relinquish my fear, trust that my Father was near my side, and then found hope in the solid truth that He would never leave me. My husband left this note on my pillow the night before surgery: *"Helo, I love you very, very much and would do anything for you. You will be in my prayers continually while in surgery. Know that you will fully recover shortly. We need you back home and will look back on this in a few years as a minor issue in our lives. Please take care of yourself and fight for us as we would fight for you. With tremendous love and adoration, Rich."*

My love for Rich became clearer than ever the night before going in for surgery. It was the end of a long day, filled with heightened emotions and preparation for what lay ahead. The night was immersed with "I love you's." We got ready to call it a night and got into bed. I did not want to sleep the time away. Instead, I wanted to stay up all night.

"Rich, please hold me and don't let go."

We fastened eyes upon each other as he gently ran his hand over my head for over an hour, repeating time and time again, "Helo, everything is going to be okay." Tears started and stopped.

I whispered, "I hope you're right."

Silence.

"I love you, Rich."

"I love you too, Helo."

We stared at each other and couldn't hold back our tears.

Then we gently embraced each other.

"Helo, we don't need to 'be together' if you simply want to be held."

At the moment, this was all we needed. He tenderly kissed me, and I kissed him back, not wanting this moment to end.

"Rich, I want to do more than just hold each other."

"Are you sure, Helo?"

I tenderly whispered, "Yes."

Slowly, we treasured each other. The question of whether this might be our last night together was unspoken yet understood. Intimacy in our marriage of decades was always beautiful, but that night its beauty was indescribable. Every single touch and affectionate moment was precious. Raw emotion on the edge brings out something rarely seen. "The way to love anything is to realize that it may be lost."[5]

Then after being together, I transparently went to a raw place that I had tried to go to with Rich several times before. Every other time he put a stop on it. This time we'd finish the conversation.

I could not believe what I was saying. "Rich, if I go, please know that I want you to remarry."

"Helo, that's not going to happen. I don't want anyone else."

Although heart wrenching, I replied, "I don't want you and the kids to spend the rest of your life without a wife and mom. I just have one triple standard. She has to genuinely love God, treasure you, and adore our children."

"Helo, you are my bar. No one can match it. I won't ever marry anyone else."

"I hope you won't have to."

"Helo, everything is going to be okay. I love you, Beautiful."

"I love you too. Please don't let go of me."

He held onto me tightly. The kind of embrace that could not be broken until morning—then we would finally let go of each other and get ready to leave. The hospital was waiting for me.

God called me to a halt, to be still, and put my life into His hands. I learned what our Heavenly Father means when He asks us to be still. I needed to rest in Him and to stop trying to anticipate what would happen. I needed to pray non-stop and understand that God was and always would be my constant companion. He was the only One who could sustain me moment by moment. I thought, *"Remember Helo, He captures every tear in His loving hands."* I fixed my eyes upon Him. "It is the Lord who goes before you. He will be with you; He will not leave you or forsake you. Do not fear or be dismayed."[6]

Chapter Three

INTO THE HANDS OF GOD

Do not tremble, do not be afraid... Is there any God besides me?
No, there is no other Rock; I know not one.

— Isaiah 44:8 —

I packed my bags the night before leaving for the hospital. It was an odd feeling to think that each task I performed that night might be the last. I showered—got dressed in sweats to simplify leaving in the morning. I cried—held on to my husband and asked him not to let go of me. We prayed again, "Please God, your child needs you now in ways that only You understand." I kept getting ready to leave for the hospital.

None of this felt real to me.

After a long night of little sleep, we left early in the morning. I didn't want to wake my sons; we had said our "I love you's" the night before. I stood outside their bedroom doors that morning, tears pouring down my cheeks.

Rich helped me into the car. I was shaking and huddling in a warm blanket. I held on to Rich's right hand, and he drove with his left. Rich is loving and brave—I needed him to be that way. I shook and wept. Everything in me wanted him to pull over, hold me, and tell me that this wasn't happening. I needed to know that there was hope—hope that I would return home to our children so I could make them dinner, hug them, hang out together, watch them trust God, go off to college, find work, get married, and have children. I wanted to grow old with my husband until we were both gray and wrinkled, talking to each other loudly because our hearing was no longer good, and repeating ourselves because in our old age we forgot things. Repeating ourselves would be okay, because hearing someone say "I love you" over and over again is incredible.

"I love you, Rich," the older me would say.

He would respond, "Eh? What did you say, good-looking? I can't hear you."

I'd repeat with a louder voice, "I love you, Rich."

He'd respond, "I love you too, Helo. That's why I tell you that over and over again."

And we would sit and watch our children play with our grandchildren who would look up at us and say, "Nana and Pop are old, but they're cute and in love." This was the dream I wanted, not the nightmare we were driving into.

Then Rich held my hand tightly and said, "Helo, I love you."

Sobbing, I whispered, "Rich, I can't hear you."

He repeated, "Helo, I love you. Everything is going to be okay."

I love Rich, but his assurances weren't enough, so he reminded me: "God is our refuge and strength, an ever-present help in trouble."[1] I threw my hands up in the air and cried out to God, "I'm heading down a road that I didn't plan. I'm shaking inside and out. Please, don't ever leave me. Take me into Your hands. My strength is wearing thin. Rain down on me Your perfect peace."

He responded, "Peace I leave with you: my peace I give you. I do not give as the world gives. Do not let your hearts be troubled and do not be afraid."[2]

After admission to the Seattle Swedish Medical Center, I had an hour-long preparatory embolization procedure in order to prevent dangerous bleeding during the surgery itself. I was rolled into the procedure room on a surgical bed with an IV drip and other attachments. The room was dark like a movie theater. High-tech equipment and flashing fluorescent lights were all around me. A video screen in front of the doctor allowed him to carefully watch what he was doing.

The doctor explained, "Helo, you are going to feel sleepy now." I was no longer aware of what was going on, so he went right to work.

A probe was inserted into a blood vessel in my groin. It traveled through the vascular network system of my body into my brain. Small particulates were inserted into the blood vessels around the brain tumor site to block the blood vessel, and end the blood supply nourishing it. Embolization minimizes risk of bleeding and also causes the tumor to lose nutrients and to shrink slightly.

In what felt like minutes, I woke up in a recovery room. The preparation was done for now, and I went back to my hospital room.

My husband stayed with me—I thought, "*This is not so bad after all.*" The preparatory procedure had been easy. We enjoyed hospital food, watched TV, and played card games. My parents stopped by to visit, and my brother-in-law, Tom, brought our two boys, Jordan and Austin, to visit me. My daughter, Lauren, was off at college and planned to visit right after the main surgery. The boys and I talked, hugged, prayed, and reassured each other that everything would be "okay." When the boys left to go home, I ached to go with them. I did not want to stay. Weeping, I held on to a family picture, reliving every cherished moment—wishing we could make more right now.

Later that evening, the hair on the left side of my head was shaved off to give the medical team access to my scalp. The hair was placed into a plastic bag. I gave it to my mom to keep. It was hard for her to look at, so she told my dad that she "threw it out." He found it later and saved it. I have yet to look at it, because I can't.

The week prior, I had asked Dr. Raisis if I should just shave my head completely bald. He'd said, "No," and told me that I was beautiful and that I shouldn't shave off all my hair, so I didn't. After surgery, I'd be able to sweep the remaining hair on my head over the left side, partially covering the scar created by opening up my skull.

Dr. Raisis compassionately shaved off my hair and placed markers on my scalp in preparation for surgery. These markers served as a surgical guide. My brain was scanned during surgery, and the markers and computer screen enabled better orientation for the operation. The majority of the surgery was performed with a microscope, its view displayed on a larger monitor.

After shaving my head, Dr. Raisis sat down and had a heartfelt conversation with my husband and me.

"Helo, you're doing well."

I was awake, alert, and responsive to questions and commands. But sitting in a hospital room, knowing what the morning would bring was unreal. Eleven days prior I had been a busy wife and mom. Now I wasn't. Continual remnants of shock consumed me.

I sat up in my hospital bed and looked around. This was nothing like home. Rich held my hand, and the serious nature of the moment overwhelmed us as Dr. Raisis described once again the procedure risks and possible complications.

"Helo, I need to make sure you fully comprehend the serious risks associated with the surgery that I'll be directing tomorrow. I know we've covered these before, and this will not be the last time we review them."

The door was shut and the room felt eerily silent. It was a private moment between Dr. Raisis, my husband, me, and God. Dr. Raisis is a compassionate doctor, the kind that makes you feel like you're the only patient he is seeing that day. Rich and I both needed him to be like that.

"Tomorrow morning you'll go in for brain tumor removal surgery. The risks include: hemorrhage, stroke, visual loss or disturbances, speech difficulties, subtotal removal of the tumor, seizures, infection, spinal fluid leak, brain infection, and death."

Riveting shock often silences the receiver. So Rich and I did not respond. Instead, I squeezed his hand harder. I cried out silently to God, more strongly than ever before.

"Helo and Rich, do you both understand the significance of how serious tomorrow's surgery is?'

Rich quietly said, "Yes."

I didn't know what to say, so I simply nodded.

Dr. Raisis looked at us and promised, "I'll take good care of you, Helo." Then he asked, "Do either one of you have any questions?"

Numb. We did not.

Dr. Raisis quietly got up from his chair, walked towards the exit, looked back at us as if to say, "Time to pray," and left the room. The door closed behind him. Now it was just me, Rich, and God. We were frightened, but not alone.

That night, a nurse gave me sleep medication so I could rest before the main surgery; I would not have slept otherwise.

I got in bed and whispered to Rich, "Do I still look beautiful to you?"

"Yes, you're always beautiful to me."

My eyes welled up with tears. "I'm scared. I don't want to leave you."

"I'm scared too, Helo, but you're going to be okay."

"Rich, know that if I go, God has my soul."

He spread another blanket over me to keep me warm and gently stroked my head until I fell asleep. Then he stayed for the whole night, sleeping on a hospital cot next to my bed.

The next morning, I put on brand-new blue hospital slippers, a surgical gown, and blue cap. Unexpectedly, I was taken to the Interventional Radiology Suite again. Dr. Raisis had observed that another major blood vessel wasn't blocked. He felt it was necessary to go back in and embolize a second time to prepare me for the main surgery. I underwent further embolization of the external carotid blood supply to the tumor in order to further reduce the bleeding risk during surgery. This was done, and there were no significant difficulties with the procedure. Recovery time following this embolization was shorter.

According to Dr. Raisis, I was finally ready for the main surgery. I lay on the gurney in a pre-operative room, waiting. The room was cold, so a nurse gave me another blanket to keep me warm. I have never tried so hard to hold back tears. Never. My family was invited in, and we had an uncanny conversation with the entire surgical team that was set to operate on my brain. This was the first time we had met them. They were compassionate, pensive, and determined.

My family was emotional, yet optimistically hopeful, as they watched the one they love go, not sure if she would come back. I was thinking the same thing. The team had to be emotionally detached—thank God they were. We signed a statement of disclosure, reviewing the risks yet again. Yes, I had heard them before a couple of times, with Dr. Raisis and Rich, but this time hearing the risks shook me hard—"vegetative state," or worse yet, "death." We all prayed fervently.

In anguish, I whispered, "God, please help me. Please hold onto me and my family. Into your hands, I now entrust myself." I distinctly remember lying on the gurney, clutching my husband's hand so tight that I was probably cutting off the circulation for both of us. I looked at my mom, dad, and husband, wishing I could freeze time—because it felt like it was evaporating. I wanted to just jump off the gurney, give them each a hug, and then run back home. But there was no turning back now. So I restrained myself and thought, *I can't do this on my own, but with God I can be brave.*

On the outside, I was trying to be strong because I needed my family to see the courageous side of me. On the inside, I was shaking like the last leaf on a tree blowing violently in a gale. My parents and husband were trying to do the same—be brave. Racing thoughts—not enough time to think—time was moving too fast. It was surreal to look at, and lock eyes with the ones I held so dear, wondering if it would be the last time I'd see them again. It was scary.

Then I whispered to God, my greatest love, "Hold on tight to me, because I need You more now than ever before." I needed to understand that God was right next to me, and that He was going to protect me forever no matter what happened. I held on tight to God—He is real.

My father then pulled Dr. Raisis aside for a moment. He desperately held back his raw emotions, put his arm around Dr. Raisis' shoulder, and implored, "This is an issue of quality of life, not quantity. If you cannot remove the entire tumor, do not perform any heroics. My daughter is a busy wife and mother." Then he reminded Dr. Raisis of the Hippocratic Oath, "Primum Non Nocere"—"First, do no harm."

Dr. Raisis answered, "Henk, I will take care of Helo as if she were my own daughter."

I finally let go of my husband's hand. I was terrified, yet it was time for me to be brave—right? Deep in my heart, I knew the only One who could give me strength. The doors to a sterile, white hall opened. I was wheeled in on the gurney, surrounded by the transfer assistants.

They gently said, "It's time to go."

I could no longer hold back tears, and neither could my family. One by one, they each kissed my forehead and said, "Helo, I love you."

I wept and softly replied, "I love you, too. Always know that God has each of us in His grip." I had so much more that I wanted to say, but there was no time left.

One of the transfer assistants repeated, "It's time to go now."

I released my husband's hand reluctantly and felt his grip even after we let go. I looked back at him as long as I could, and whispered again, "I love you." We turned a corner, and then I couldn't see my family anymore.

The heavy doors to the main surgical hallway opened. I felt a swish of cold air pass by. On either side of the gurney were two men dressed in blue—the transfer assistants. I looked up at their faces; they looked determined and intense. They were moving me steadily and quickly. The gurney was strong, with metal railings, and felt like it was on ice skates as it glided across the floor. At that point, I noticed the starched, crisp, white sheets that covered me. The hallway was bright. White. Wide. I felt like I was in a tunnel, staring up at the lights on the ceiling.

I told myself, *"I'm leaving my family only for a little while. Do not look at what you might lose; look at all that you have. You are in the skilled hands of an incredible neurosurgeon, and the hands of God are incomparably stronger."*

The gurney turned again, then stopped, and another set of doors whooshed open. We passed through. The doors shut behind me and made a loud, mechanical click that I will never forget. *I was shaking inside.*

We had reached the main surgical suite. The room was bright, white, sterile, and cold. It smelled cleaner than home. I was now surrounded by more machinery than I had ever seen before, above and around me. Clicking. Flashing lights. Odd sounds. Wires. Tubes.

Everyone was dressed in blue and busy. I was lined up right next to a massive table. A loud ratcheting noise sounded as they locked the operating table in place. More loud noise. The gurney brakes were locked. A man stood right next to my side. He grabbed the gurney's railing and a loud "swish and click" sounded as it was pulled down. I thought, "*This place is noisy.*" At the same time wires, tubes, and equipment were moved away from me. Then I heard them say, "Okay, Helo, we are going to move you now."

It felt like I was enveloped in a white, starchy hammock resting on top of a plastic board. Three people surrounded me—one at my head, one at my feet, and one by my side. They said in cadence, "One, two," and on "three," moved my body onto the stiff operating table. They quickly adjusted my positioning, moved the sheets, secured parts of my body down with straps, pulled down a portion of my gown and brought back wires, tubes, and machinery. I heard more beeping and clicking.

I heard water running in the sink. I saw someone assisting Dr. Raisis with his gloves. He had on a mask, the whole surgical garb, and a light on his head. He looked so different than he had in his office. I was being poked with needles, including an IV put into my inner elbow. A cuff was wrapped around my arm. Wires were attached to my upper torso with sticky tabs. Tubes were placed in my nose and at first it felt suffocating, as if air was being forced in, but there was no time to argue about their placement. This was all happening so fast. I'm thinking, "*Okay, now I know this is real.*"

The anesthesiologist said, "Helo, you're going to sleep now."

Tears rolled down my face as I looked up and locked eyes with Dr. Raisis. He looked at me and said, "I am going to take good care of you, Beautiful."

I gave him a quick smile and whispered, "Thanks." I thought to myself, "*I love you, Rich. I love you Lauren, Jordan, Austin, Dad, Mom...*" I wanted to list everyone that I loved, but time was running out. My whispers became faint. "I love you, God." The cold and sterile room began to look fuzzy, and I fell asleep. That's what anesthesia does.

I drifted off, surrounded by the expert medical team assembled by Dr. Raisis. He had even asked his primary assistant to come back from vacation for my surgery because of its complexity. He approximated that the surgery would last around seven hours, and his plan was to stay for the entire surgery, as his protocol is to "never leave the patient's side and do not take breaks."

The brain is the most complex organ that God created. It orchestrates every function. Damage to it can cause damage to any of the body's capabilities. And it sits, inside a relatively thin protective shell. That shell had to be opened.

The final preparation for surgery was delicate and methodical. A plastic tube was inserted down the back of my throat, through the windpipe, and into the bronchial tubes of my lungs. Machines helped me breathe. Then a central venous line for administering drugs and an arterial line for monitoring blood pressure were put in place. A catheter was used to manage and control the fluid surrounding the brain. My body was securely strapped down, and my head was fixed into a head holder and positioned for a left frontotemporal craniotomy (cutting through the skull). The left side of my head was then prepped with Betadine and draped in a sterile manner.

Dr. Raisis stood with the surrounding team, held his right hand open and said, "Scalpel."

A twelve-inch incision in the shape of a large reverse question mark was cut into my scalp. The incision began above my left ear and extended toward the back of my head. The skin flap covering the skull was elevated. This exposed the temporalis muscle, which was then incised and elevated. The goal was to not injure the nerve that goes to the face.

The bone had to be cut open without disturbing the brain. Four holes were drilled into my skull. (The drill has a sensor that determines when it should stop so as not to hit the brain.) All bone fragments were saved in a sterile container. Then a saw was carefully used to cut out a bone flap from my skull. All bone dust was preserved to be used later when my skull was closed back up.

At this point, the brain was exposed, but the outermost membrane, the dura that envelopes and bathes the brain and spinal chord with cerebrospinal fluid, had not yet been cut. The fluid had to be preserved by plugging the dura to prevent leakage. Tubes were put in the area, and suction was applied.

There, on the operating table, I had an unexpected generalized seizure which was extremely concerning, because I was under general anesthesia at the time. Dr. Raisis was not sure what triggered the seizure because the dura had not yet been opened. I received medication, and the seizure abated. My brain initially appeared swollen but then settled down and began to pulsate. I was given more medication, and doctors induced hyperventilation to treat the swelling.

The dura was cut open and pulled out of the way to expose the brain. At this point, the grey matter of the brain, where the intellectual functions are housed, was exposed.

The tumor was deeply hidden, and the doctor had to carefully make his way through my brain. To access the tumor for removal, parts of the brain had to be moved out of the way without doing harm to the sensitive structures that regulate and monitor all functions. Dr. Raisis retracted another lobe of the brain. With careful microsurgical techniques, using a binocular operating microscope, he exposed the tumor.

Numerous large blood vessels fed the tumor; Dr. Raisis thought they looked like a "snake pit of blood vessels." He carefully cauterized the vessels to stop blood flow. He was determined to do it right the first time, because if he didn't, scar tissue would form, making the tumor difficult to go after again. Proceeding slowly and meticulously, he eventually got completely around the soft, whitish-gray tumor. He was able to remove the tumor in totality. He then inspected the surrounding area of the brain and removed any small tumor remnants.

The ugly tumor was placed in a jar, and the lid was shut.

The area of the brain where the tumor had been housed was irrigated with copious amounts of saline and antibiotic solution. There was no more bleeding. The dura was closed in a watertight fashion, and the bone flap was replaced. It was secured to the skull using titanium plates and two-millimeter screws. The preserved bone dust and chips were used to fill the area where the bone had been cut. This was to help the skull heal. The doctors took care to eliminate any space between the brain and skull, and then closed the temporalis muscle. The scalp was closed with staples; sterile dressing was applied and wrapped around my head. All needles and sponges were accounted for at the termination of this procedure to make sure that none had been left inside my head. Dr. Raisis believed that I tolerated the procedure well, and I was transported to the Postoperative Anesthesia Care Unit in "good" condition.

I cannot imagine what it was like for my family to sit and wait in a private waiting room for seven long hours—maybe the wait felt suffocating. It was a blessing that I didn't know. The anesthesiologist finally came out to tell my family that the surgery had gone exceptionally well, and he was pleased with the outcome. Dr. Raisis would provide more details. He came out twenty minutes later with a smile of relief on his face, exclaiming, "I removed the entire tumor!" Using the latest technology, he showed my family photographs of the surgery, including one of the tumor in my brain and then in a jar.

Shortly after the operation, I was moved from the surgical recovery room to the Intensive Care Unit. Two hours passed after surgery before my family could see me. With my husband and parents present, Dr. Raisis attempted to wake me up from the anesthesia. He wanted to confirm that I could still speak, see, respond to simple questions, and move my arms and legs. This was typical procedure for him to establish a baseline after surgery.

He brought me to semi-consciousness. I responded groggily.

Dr. Raisis asked, "What's your name?"

I responded, "Helo."

"Helo, do you know where you are?"

"In the hospital."

"How old are you?'

"I don't know."

"Helo, count to ten." I did. Slowly.

"Count backwards from ten to one."

I succeeded.

"Helo, how much is eight plus seven?"

Quietly, I mumbled, "Fifteen."

He gave me simple instructions: "Helo, move your left arm, move your right arm, raise your left leg and your right leg." And I did. Barely.

Dr. Raisis examined my eye movements and the reaction of my pupils. He was satisfied that everything was intact and the surgery hadn't caused any loss of function or serious harm. Dr. Raisis was very pleased, and my family was extremely thankful.

Now we had to work towards recovery.

Some physicians do not check a patient right after major surgery, believing it is better to allow them to rest and recover overnight before conducting simple tests, but Dr. Raisis wanted tests done as soon as possible to give him, and my family, peace of mind. Had we waited until the next morning, there would have been no reassuring response. My family was excited about the visual evidence that the surgery had succeeded; it provided a sense of comfort during the weeks ahead.

Moments of reprieve and hope surface during trials. For example, my family found peace shortly after surgery. It was God's way of blessing and strengthening them so they could persevere. The tumor was benign. The procedure had gone well. This was a trial that my family could manage. I was, after all, going to be home within a week.

Chapter Four

THE LONGEST SIX DAYS EVER

Always remember that the future comes one day at a time.
— Dean Acheson[1] —

My neurosurgeon, Dr. Raisis, had been in practice for twenty-nine years, yet on only one other occasion had he extracted a tumor like mine. A study of the tumor later revealed the type: a microcystic meningioma. It is a rare tumor—only one in two million—and has a particularly nasty trait. Removing it from my brain was like touching poison ivy, causing my brain to swell dramatically. As a result, it wasn't until several hours after surgery that my trial intensified and serious complications developed. In spite of the fact that God gifted Dr. Raisis with the extraordinary ability to take care of me, the unthinkable began.

I was not going home in six days.

My brain began to swell. As the pressure on it increased, I became less and less responsive to outside stimuli. There was an intense discussion as to the best course of action. The doctors thought about removing the portion of my skull that had just been reattached. The intent was to relieve the pressure. The bone plate would be preserved by placing it under the skin near my stomach for later use. This was a dangerous option because the pressure was so high that a portion of my brain could, potentially, burst out of my skull.

Early one day when my dad came to visit me in the ICU, he checked my reflexes and my pupils as usual. He did this daily at random. He opened my eyes and discovered that my left pupil was enlarged, indicating that the pressure on the brain stem was horrendously high. It meant that my brain was going into herniation, which is catastrophic like a major heart attack, only it's the brain having an attack and entering failure mode. He became alarmed. The on-call intensivist just happened to be doing rounds and walked into my room to check on me. My dad immediately told the intensivist what he'd just seen.

The intensivist asked, "Are you sure?"

My dad confirmed.

The intensivist opened my left eye and quickly checked. The dilating pupil signified that the pressure on the brain was dangerously high and needed to be brought down immediately, or I could die within minutes. The crash cart was pulled in. Dr. Raisis was urgently called to the scene. He ran in and ordered my dad to leave the room.

My dad, the physician, was petrified.

Within seconds, a tube was quickly inserted down my throat for intubation. A respirator was connected to breathe for me rapidly, purposefully causing me to hyperventilate. The intent was to reduce the pressure in my brain. Medications were quickly administered: steroids to reduce swelling and diuretics to intentionally induce dehydration. Then my entire body was placed between two plasto-fabric ice blankets from head to toe—inducing hypothermia. The goal was to slow my body's metabolism and decrease the brain swelling. All of this happened within minutes; time was of the essence.

Dr. Raisis ordered further adjustments and a brain CT scan to see if anything was helping. The results showed that my brain was still swollen. I remained in ice sheets for three days. The induced hypothermia was monitored to gage core temperature to guard against heart arrhythmias and skin breakdown. If the ice sheets did their job, they would be removed, and my body would carefully enter the re-warming phase.

Thank God my dad checked my eyes at that exact moment. Thank God the intensivist walked in at the right time. By the time the machines could have caught the problem, and alarms sounded, it would've been too late. No vital signs would've been left to measure, because I would've been gone. Thank God that waiting worked, and no further deterioration occurred.

However, I was not out of the woods yet. A new ominous worry took hold; in addition to increased pressure in my brain because of swelling, there was the possibility of simultaneous postoperative bleeding. A scan showed no bleeding, but indicated that the swelling was as bad as it could be. The hematologist took a precautionary step to monitor my condition and administered additional blood products to minimize bleeding risk.

Medications, including propofol, and machines kept me in a comatose state to allow my brain to rest. Machines, tubes, and wires helped my lungs breathe, monitored my heart and blood flow, provided nutrients, and kept my bladder empty, among other things, so my brain could concentrate on healing rather than on directing and controlling regular bodily functions. Later, my brain went into its own coma and medications were no longer necessary to put my brain into this state.

If I could think, I would have thought, *"Angels of Heaven, please surround me."*

The ICU team at the Swedish Medical Center was phenomenal. Multiple nurses were dedicated to me, and my family got to know them well. My husband and parents stayed at my side continually, not knowing what would happen next. Rich kissed me every day while I was in the ICU, even though it was hard for him to get to my cheek because of all the wires and tubes from the life-support machinery. He held my hand and talked to me as if I could hear him, even though I didn't respond. This was a unique conversation for a wife and husband to have; typically, the wife does most of the talking.

If I could've told him what I needed to hear him say, it would've been, "Tell me how much you love me and the kids. Say that you don't want to let me go. Tell me to pull Jesus by my side so that I'll find hope and not give up. Promise me that we'll always be together, and tell me that I am beautiful inside and out. Pray out loud so that we can both hear our conversation with our Father. Remind me that God will never leave my side, yours, or our children's. Tell me that you understand that no matter what, that even if I become severely disabled or vegetative, we'll be okay. Say that if I take my final breath and angels close my eyes, you'll remember that our family is in the grip of His comfort and we will all one day be reunited in Heaven. Continue to keep me company—don't let go of my hand. And if I go, don't you cry when I'm gone. I'm in His hands, where I belong, where the afflictions of this world will hurt no more."

After five days in the hospital, my family was emotionally drained and physically exhausted. They came up with a plan to be on alternating shifts to stay by my side. My parents stayed at a hotel a few blocks away from the hospital; they visited me each morning and stayed through lunch. My husband arrived around the lunch hour after spending time with the boys at home and stayed until late in the evening after the nursing shift change. Rich never left without tucking me in and saying, "I love you, Helo. Goodnight."

The unthinkable continued. On my sixth day in the ICU, the oxygen monitor sounded an alarm at two a.m. I was turning blue because one of my lungs had collapsed. My oxygen saturation levels had dropped to fifty percent. Normal levels hover between ninety and one hundred percent. A nurse called a *Code Blue*. She grabbed equipment to pump air into my lungs until doctors arrived. Every available doctor on staff was called into my room to rescue me. Their valiant efforts kept me alive.

My family learned about this incident in the morning. It had happened on the first evening that my husband had not stayed in the hospital through the entire night. He felt terrible to have finally gone home to spend the night with our children, only to learn that he had almost lost his beloved wife and best friend. As much as this troubled him, he knew that he must continue to trust God and the physicians to take care of me.

"I love the Lord, for He heard my voice; He heard my cry for mercy Because He turned his ear to me, I will call on Him as long as I live."

— Psalm 116:1–2

Later that day, a pulmonologist was called in to check on my lungs and found irregularity in my breathing. Turns out, I had pneumonia. Medications were in place to do their best to keep my lungs undisturbed, but the pulmonologist suspected that there was a plug in one of my lungs that could cause coughing despite the drugs in my system. When the brain shakes too hard, as with a concussion, it is bad. If the brain is already compromised because of massive swelling, like mine was, even coughing just once would shake my brain. This would increase the pressure in my brain, elevating the risk of herniation that could cause death. Within seconds, the pulmonologist inserted a suction tube into my intubation tube and removed the mucous plug. This prevented life-threatening coughing. The timing was perfect; I believe that God was again protecting me.

Dr. Raisis visited me daily in the ICU, each morning and evening. He often ran a key along the bottom of my foot, checking to see if I had regained any level of consciousness, and asked, "Helo, are you in there?" When a newborn's feet are scratched underneath, the toes curl in because the brain is not fully developed. A healthy adult brain responds to a key run along the bottom of a foot by telling the toes to curl out. The trauma that my brain faced kept it from communicating with my feet, and my toes responded to the key by curling in, like a newborn's.

After doing this check, Dr. Raisis would firmly tap his fingers against my sternum, asking again, "Helo, are you in there?" He received no response. God, the Great Physician knew that I was in there; my neurosurgeon needed to check and see. Everyone was asking, "When will the brain swelling subside?" My brain had inflated precariously, and its midline had shifted. Doctors wondered if I had suffered a stroke because the left side of my body was completely unresponsive and immobile. Would there be a full recovery? Could I go home? Or would I spend the rest of my life in a nursing home? The doctors could write no timetable or map of recovery for me—*only God knew.*

My husband, children, and extended family experienced incomprehensible stress and sorrow as they watched their loved one in a state of affliction. Hope and non-stop prayer sustained them. No loving husband ever wants to lose his wife, no child can comprehend the potential of losing a parent, and no parent wants to contemplate the idea of outliving his or her child. Trauma like this initiates tears; guarded optimism helps to soften the pain.

Contemplation of my death at such a young age pulled my family to a place of grasping onto hope, despite everything they had recently seen. My husband asked everyone to reflect on this Bible verse "…weeping may stay for the night, but rejoicing comes in the morning."[2] My family endured watching me on life support, hoping and praying that tomorrow would be better.

> "Though the mountains be shaken and the hills be removed, yet my unfailing love for you will not be shaken, nor my covenant of peace be removed," says the Lord, who has compassion on you."
>
> — Isaiah 54:10

A week and an half into my ICU stay, the wounds from my surgery had started to heal, and Dr. Raisis removed the gauze and staples from my head. I remained motionless. Doctors and family still had no idea if or when I would wake up; so once again, they had to be patient and wait. The intensive treatment to reduce the swelling was beginning to pay off. The doctor's knew this because my pupil size was becoming more equal on both the right and left sides.

Finally, a few days later, I opened my eyes and was able to follow some simple commands. I was in danger, but I was still in there. My family was thrilled. Perhaps we were on our way to getting off of this seemingly unending path of discouragement.

> "You will be secure, because there is hope; you will look about you and take rest in safety."
>
> — Job 11:18

God's healing power demonstrated itself in small yet hopeful ways. Together, with God's lead, my family and I began to conquer the pain and suffering.

Rich and my dad attempted to communicate with me, although I could not speak while intubated. They'd ask me to give a thumbs-up if the answer was "yes" and a thumbs-down if the answer was "no." This worked well, though communication was limited as I tired easily, was intensely weak, and could fall asleep at any moment. *I don't remember this.*

As I became more responsive, the breathing apparatus was finally removed and a feeding tube to my stomach was placed in my nose. A dietician then came on board to direct my nutrition. Eating was not simple. My dad, the rehabilitation doctor, asked if a speech pathologist could conduct a swallowing evaluation as a baseline and then repeat it to monitor my progress. I abhorred the feeding tube, threw a tantrum, and tried to yank it out of my nose. My dad restrained me. I love my father and always will, but I did not appreciate being treated like a two-year old.

In fairness to my dad, I needed the intervention because the majority of my functioning was not even at the level of a newborn baby. The hospital staff then stepped in, put cuff restraints on my fragile, yet stubborn, wrists, and attached me to my bed railings. I had absolutely no interest in being anchored to my bed.

I still despised the feeding tube. If I took enough food by mouth, the feeding tube would be removed. My type-A personality displayed itself, and I insisted upon extra food at once. I had ordinarily been thought of as polite, but not then. I quickly demonstrated that sometimes politeness can be replaced by determination and frustration. *This too can work!* The next day, the annoying feeding tube was disconnected.

Two days later, I had a follow-up swallowing evaluation. Relief set in for my family and medical staff as I started to display improvement. I began working on food intake. Applesauce was brought to my mouth with the help of the speech pathologist. I sat bolt upright, and with every swallow, I had to put my chin down to my chest. This was not a natural way to eat, nor was it comfortable. I did not enjoy eating in this complicated manner. Two days later, my diet was promoted to palatable milkshakes. I had a strong preference for chocolate.

It's hard to imagine how often we take such simple abilities as swallowing for granted. Being able to eat, even with a considerable amount of help, was a blessing. Dr. Raisis wanted to keep me in the ICU as long as possible, to prevent future possible complications. But my dad was focused on something different. He was ready for me to move forward with rehabilitation, and wanted to put the ICU behind us. *Everyone did.*

I was started on basic occupational and physical therapy while I was in the ICU. My dad, an experienced rehabilitation medicine physician, wanted to make sure that I did not suffer complications such as Achilles tendon shortening, reduced joint range of motion, and muscle atrophy from prolonged immobility in the ICU.

These complications could likely be prevented by early intervention. As I became somewhat more responsive, my dad wanted to harness my future progress through appropriate therapy with sensory input to stimulate brain function. I tended to neglect my left side and this needed to change. I had to relearn how to feed myself and how to move in bed. It would have been nice if I could participate in getting dressed, but it would be a long time before I was able to.

First, I worked on my balance just to sit up in bed. With help on both sides, I sat up. The physical therapist instructed, "Now, Helo, dangle your feet at the end of the bed. Sit for just two minutes."

I cried, "I cannot do it." My body slumped over, and my husband and physical therapist caught me. With help, I sat up again.

Now sitting on the edge of the bed, my physical therapist insisted, "Get up Helo, and stand."

I hesitated, and then mumbled, "I can't."

She needed to be firm. "Helo, stand up, now."

"I'm scared!" I saw two of everything and the walls looked crooked.

"Helo, Rich and I will hold onto you. We will not let you fall. Stand up."

I did, slowly. *It was so hard.* I stood on my feet, with others holding onto me tightly, for just a few seconds. Without them, I would've dropped to the floor.

"See, Helo, you can do it. We are not going to let go of you. Now try to lift your right leg and take one step."

Really? "I cannot stand anymore. I feel weak." I was shaking and felt like flopping to the ground.

"Okay, Helo, that's enough for today."

Rich and the therapist held onto me tight as I sat back down. They lifted my legs and helped me turn to lie back in bed. I sobbed, "God help me. Please help me." And then I reminded myself, "*Each step taken forward is one step away from this affliction and one step closer to conquering it. Don't give up, Helo.*"

I'd been in therapy for five minutes and had nothing left to give. The therapist determined that I was done for the day, and I quickly fell asleep. Five minutes was nowhere near the three hour goal, but more would come in the days and weeks ahead.

My dad felt that the prognosis for my full recovery with occupational, speech, and physical therapy was good, but wanted to make sure that this wasn't simply a father's wishful thinking. He also didn't want to burden the ICU staff with asking them to introduce rehabilitation therapy so early on, before knowing for sure that it was the right thing to do. He requested a second objective opinion from Dr. Margaret Forgette, a partner in his former medical practice. She conducted a rehabilitation evaluation to assess the prognosis for recovery. She confirmed that the prognosis for recovery was good. My dad was encouraged by her optimism. One day I should be able to walk, talk, think, and function again following extensive rehab.

The care coordinator commented that she'd never seen rehabilitation medicine involved so early on in the ICU. In retrospect, I realize that the early rehab intervention gave me a head start on inpatient rehabilitation, without the typical complications from a prolonged ICU stay. Although I had moments when I didn't like the early initiation of therapy directed by my dad, he prepared me for Dr. David Tempest, a rehabilitation medicine specialist, who would soon direct the lengthy process of inpatient rehabilitative care.

As the lead physician, Dr. Raisis made the final decision on when to move me out of the ICU. With my discharge from the ICU forthcoming, my husband requested that the ICU staff wash my hair. This request surprised them because washing a patient's hair in the ICU was rare. In fact, these nurses had to consult with other nurses to determine how to proceed. They searched for appropriate supplies. A small plastic tub was placed upon a towel underneath my head. A nurse gently took my sleepy head into her hands while a second nurse helped wash my hair with warm soapy water. I was completely unaware that this was going on because exhaustion made me sleep up to twenty-one hours a day, but my husband wanted me to feel kept up and beautiful.

Soon, we would travel to the rehabilitation unit at the Swedish Medical Center.

Chapter Five

THE QUEST FOR REHABILITATION

Our greatest weakness lies in giving up. The most certain way to succeed is always to try just one more time.

— Thomas A. Edison —

Three weeks following surgery, I was exhausted. Almost two and a half years later, I asked Dr. Raisis why I was so tired and fragile back then. He told me, "Even though you appeared to be resting while in a coma, your body was focusing all of its energy on recovery. Your brain endured a lot of trauma and needed equal rest time to recover."

After finally waking up in the ICU, I looked at myself in the mirror and was shocked. I stared at the extensive black and blue bruises on my arms and neck; they disturbed me. And I silently wondered, *"Who is that person in the mirror? What happened to me?"* They were the result of life-supporting IVs. The discoloration eventually went away, but the bruises simply confirmed a small portion of what I'd been through in the ICU. I was no longer attached to machines, and I was alive. For this, I am thankful.

The challenge of pressing onward through continued recovery is often far more intimidating than the suffering initially inflicted. But when I accepted the challenge of suffering and backed away from giving up, I found hope—over and over again.

Upon being discharged from the ICU, I was transferred to the inpatient rehabilitation department at the Swedish Medical Center via a disabled patient van. Although the trip is less than a mile, the process of leaving the ICU and transferring to the rehab unit took more than two hours. It was both physically and emotionally taxing, yet I was excited to begin the rehab process. This was the first time in three weeks that I felt fresh air as I was wheeled outside. *Fresh air is amazing.*

My stay in the rehab unit was originally scheduled for three weeks but was extended to five. I was placed in room 627, the one closest to the nurses' station. My dad found that eerie—he'd worked in that very rehab unit for twenty-five years and treated many patients in room 627. It was surreal for him to visit me there. One day, I gave my dad a big hug and told him, "Now I know clearly what kind of work you've been doing for all these years. You are exceptional at it."

The rehab unit was very different from the ICU, and for good reason. The rooms were softer—laid out more like a nice hotel than a hospital. The halls were filled with other people in recovery, and the atmosphere was one of hope. It wasn't home, and I still was not where I wanted to be, but perhaps I was well on my way. It was better.

I once was an active and fit person. During rehab with my father, I struggled with taking baby steps to get better. *Learning how to do almost everything over again was not easy.* I was to start physical, occupational, and speech therapy with a goal of three hours of therapy sessions every day. This seemed overly ambitious to my husband. During the last day in the ICU, my major accomplishment had been getting out of bed once, and that had required significant assistance. In that session, I'd stood up with help and attempted to take one step. *Moving my feet had felt impossible.* Supported on both sides, I'd turned around and returned to the bed with tears of frustration. I could see the door less than five feet away and wanted to walk towards it. *Not that day.*

I repeatedly cried out, "God, please help me to walk again."

After moving to the rehabilitation unit, the first official day of inpatient rehab began. During the first session, I worked with the speech therapist. She asked many questions to assess my cognitive functioning and reasoning skills. This would be repeated on a daily basis to evaluate progress.

When the physical therapist came in, I struggled to get out of bed and became discouraged. Trying to stand and then walk by myself was basically impossible. With help, I was able to take two steps; then I broke down sobbing on the border of helplessness. I shouted to the physical therapist, "I am done!"

I didn't know if God or anyone else was even listening to me. Why did I have to learn how to do everything over again? I was overwhelmed, but giving up was not an option.

"From the ends of the earth will I cry out unto thee, when my heart is overwhelmed: lead me to the rock that is higher than I."

— Psalm 61:2, KJV

My complaints didn't convince the rehab staff to give in to my feeble attempts to quit, because they were not going to quit either. God never left my side—so I kept seeking hope. I could breathe on my own now. I wanted to stand and walk again. *I just wanted to go home.* Time for me to step aside from what *I wanted*, and allow God to show me His will.

Late in the afternoon on my first day of rehab, Rich touched my shoulders and woke me up from a long nap. I still spent more time sleeping than staying awake.

"Helo, time to get up, a doctor is on his way to see you," Rich told me.

"No please, not another one. What's this one for?" I complained.

"You need to be evaluated to see if you can continue to stay here in rehab," Rich said.

"So I might get to go home now?"

"No, Helo, they need to see if you should stay here or move to a long-term care facility."

"What's that?"

"A nursing home, Helo," Rich quietly replied. I could tell by the look on his face that he was a bit sad.

"A nursing home?" Now I was angry and exasperated. "I am not going to a nursing home. Help me get ready to see the doctor."

Rich helped me sit up in bed, put on my hospital robe, and then he swept my hair back. Moments later, there was a knock on the door.

"Helo, I am Dr. 'Smith'. Can I come in?"

"Yes, doctor," I responded.

In walked a psychiatrist dressed in a navy suit, crisp white shirt, and decorated tie, carrying a clipboard. He asked Rich to leave the room, closed the door behind him and sat down in a chair across from me. He had a calm yet inquisitive look on his face. I held my head up, looked at the doctor, and felt like I was about to face a medical inquisition.

And so began the flood of questions: "Do you understand why you are here? How do you feel? Do you want to stay here? Can you do this?" I responded slowly with, "I know why I am here, but I don't want to be—I'd rather be home, I feel trapped inside of my body because it does not work like it is supposed to. But I am determined, and by God's grace I will pull through."

Thankfully, after what felt like a draining hour of countless questions and delayed answers, I passed the psychiatric evaluation and it was determined that I was "emotionally ready" to continue with rehabilitation therapy. The doctor got up and before he left the room, he looked back at me, and said, "Helo, you will get to stay here until you are strong enough to go home." The door closed behind him, and I thought to myself, "*Just give me a moment everybody. I am fragile, but God is going to keep me strong.*"

Rich came back into the room; I did my best to smile and whispered, "I'm going to get to stay." He said, "I love you, Helo," gave me a hug, tucked me back in bed, kissed my forehead, and then I fell asleep—again.

Towards the end of the second day of therapy, I was not making progress. I wanted to stay in bed and sleep all day. The rehab staff wanted me to engage in three hours of daily therapy, and my husband encouraged me, to no avail. Finally, Dr. Tempest ran tests concluding that I had pneumonia. This was my second bout of pneumonia in two weeks. The silver lining—a day of reprieve. Physical therapy stopped temporarily for twenty-four hours. *I needed rest.*

Therapy resumed again shortly after my pneumonia diagnosis. At this point, it took multiple people to sit me up. I was a collapsing, frustrated, easily distracted, and annoyed Raggedy Ann doll. I wanted to sleep constantly. I needed help sitting on a portable toilet, cleaning myself, and pulling up my underwear. This was humiliating. Oh, but this was only the tip of the humiliation iceberg!

Weekly team conferences were held with an interdisciplinary team in a private conference room, which felt like a corporate boardroom to me. I sat silently in a wheelchair at these conferences and often felt like falling asleep. *Traumatized brains do this.* Sessions were directed by Dr. David Tempest, the lead rehabilitation physician. Also in attendance were physical, occupational, and speech therapists; a psychologist, a nurse, and my family.

I remember feeling like a puppet under evaluation: "Can she stand, walk, talk, hold a spoon, swallow, sit up, wash her hair, use the restroom, and raise her hand?" Discussion and determination continued. I wondered if I still needed strings to help me function like a puppet or if I'd ever be able to perform tasks on my own again.

My medical progress was documented by Dr. Tempest and therapists, as were any "barriers to achievement of goals." Doctors revised those goals weekly and evaluated whether I was finally ready to leave the rehab unit. Discharge disposition was the goal we were working toward, but week after week, my ability to leave was ruled out by the medical team.

I was determined to press on, and so was my family and medical staff. I learned that frustration blanketed by hope turns into determination. I told myself, *"Don't quit, Helo. God is never going to leave you."* I chose to persevere because I knew that God would not let go of me, and the battle of moving forward, was not for me to fight alone. I clung onto this truth to get me through the moments of feeling beaten.

"What lies behind us and what lies ahead of us are tiny matters compared to what lies within us."

—Ralph Waldo Emerson

I could open my mouth only about a quarter of an inch because of temporalis muscle atrophy due to the surgery. My surgeon was concerned that my mouth would lock shut, so I had to squeeze a rubber ball into my mouth to stretch it open multiple times every day. I took a soft, blue, malleable, rubber ball filled with sand and squeezed as much of it as I could into my mouth. It was a workout for my mouth and fingers. It hurt my jaws. I was supposed to keep it in my mouth for as long as possible several times a day. Then I had to carefully slip it back through my clenched teeth, without popping it and getting a mouthful of sand.

Rich sometimes asked me, "How does it feel, Helo?" It's hard to respond with a rubber ball in your mouth—so I just groaned, did my best to mumble, and shook my head instead of talking. This made Rich smile. *It did not make me happy.* I got to stick this silly ball of sand in my mouth for several months. A quarter of an inch turned into half an inch, half an inch turned into three-quarters, and pretty soon (within a few months) I could open my mouth with ease. Not like I used to before surgery—but I could still open it.

When eating, I had trouble dipping a spoon into the applesauce. My hand shook, felt weak, and didn't feel like it belonged to me. I thought, *"Time to focus Helo."* I put the spoon in the cup of applesauce. Now the next challenge was lifting it steadily toward my mouth without spilling it everywhere. I looked down at the spoon and thought, *"Helo, feed yourself."* Shaking, but attempting to keep my hand steady, I brought the spoon to my lips, but opening my mouth was hard. I couldn't open it all the way. The spoon entered my mouth but not all of its contents made it in—so I slobbered as the remnants dripped down the sides of my face. I kept thinking, *"This is not how I am supposed to eat. I'm embarrassed…but the applesauce tastes so good."* After struggling for awhile, others helped me finish eating.

I was unable to wash my own hair, so a therapist showed me how to wash my hair by doing it for me. Days later, I washed my hair with help, but when I was told to open the shampoo bottle, I couldn't. So the therapist opened it for me, told me to open my hand, and poured shampoo into my palm. I looked at the shampoo and tried to lift my trembling hand to my head, but it didn't work and my hand fell to my lap. Once again, I had to rely on someone else to help me wash my hair. Humiliated, I felt like screaming. But didn't.

One day, a therapist walked into my hospital room. "Time to get undressed, Helo."

"Am I going to take a shower?"

"Yes, and I will help you."

She watched me get out of bed, helped me get undressed, sit in a plastic chair in the shower, told me not to stand—I might slip and fall—pointed out the shampoo and soap sitting on a shelf, and showed me the emergency call button.

"Where are you going?" I asked.

"I'm going to step outside the room and you're going to wash your hair by yourself today."

"I can't."

"Time to start learning how. You can do it, Helo. Press the emergency call button if you need anything. I will check back on you in a little while."

She turned on the water, showed me how to adjust it, and closed the shower curtain.

I sat and sobbed with water pouring over my face. It felt like half an hour went by. I washed only the ends of my hair because my frail arms couldn't lift my hands to the top of my head.

The therapist came back in and opened the shower curtain.

"How did it go, Helo?"

Shivering a little, I said, "I'm clean now—well, most of me is."

"Good, here's a towel."

I dried off the parts of me that I could reach and she helped me with the rest. By this time Rich was in the room. He helped me get dressed and tucked me in bed.

During therapy, I walked the hallways daily, but walking was difficult early on without my physical therapist on one side, my husband on the other, and a walker in front of me. Without their assistance, I would've fallen to the floor. I also had a tendency to walk into walls. I remember telling myself, *"Do not to walk into the walls, Helo, because it might be embarrassing and you might bonk your head."* It had been through enough already.

The physical therapist asked me to hold my head up high and focus on something a few steps ahead: a doorknob, a picture on the wall, or a window. "Look straight ahead, Helo. Helo! Focus on your goal. You only have four more steps to go. You can do it, Helo." Walking had never been so hard, and I felt overwhelmed. *I asked God to walk with me every step of the way.* Then I sat down and rested. Sometimes a wheelchair was brought to me to go back to my room. Other times, I rested, got back up, focused, and made my way back to my room with my husband on one side and my physical therapist on the other.

For physical therapy, I was instructed to sit up straight on a large table covered with an exercise mat. The table was so big that other patients were working on opposite ends of it. Rich stood by and watched.

The physical therapist encouraged, "Okay Helo, show me that you can sit."

I did, looked back, and grumbled, "This is harder than sitting in a chair because there is no back behind me."

"Sitting this way is good for you to learn."

"Yeah, but it makes me feel tired."

"It will also make you stronger, Helo."

"Okay, I am done sitting now."

"Good. Now it's time for you to stand up."

I did and thought, *"Can I go back to my room now?"* This was obviously not an option. *"Humph."*

The therapist then said, "Helo, here's a big blue exercise ball. Now I'm going to stand back and I want you raise it up and throw it to me."

"*Really?*" I thought to myself, "*This ought to be easy. I've played in the park with my children when they were little. I can do this. No problem.*"

But it wasn't. Holding onto the ball tight, without dropping it, wasn't simple—I threw it a couple of feet and watched it bounce. "Can we please stop now? I need to sit down again."

The therapist retrieved the ball and countered, "No Helo, I am going to throw it to you now and you are going to catch it."

"*Really?*"

She tossed it a few feet toward me. I watched it roll gently past.

She looked at me and urged, "Go get the ball, Helo."

I don't like to play fetch often and I'm not a puppy—but I had three children and a husband to go home to, and I couldn't wait to play in the backyard with them. So despite a longing to quit listening to commands regarding ball retrieval, I tried as hard as I could. Sometimes I would just kick the ball a few feet and the therapist reminded me that my lazy response was *not* what she was looking for me to do.

After several times of throwing it a few feet back and forth to each other, the physical therapist and I were done playing with the big blue ball. Learning how to throw, bounce, and catch a ball is challenging when your brain has no idea what you're trying to do. After weeks of therapy, playing ball became easier and I learned to appreciate the skill.

My next task was to go into a make-believe house area in rehab and walk up and down fabricated stairs. Lifting my legs to walk up each step was challenging. I paused and rested often. Turning around to come down four steps was daunting. Sometimes I stopped midway and sobbed. But I didn't give up. After my walking adventure, I was asked to get in and out of a pretend metal car. I'd never thought something like this would be so difficult, and being patient was tough. But God showed me over and over again how patient He is with me.

Weeks later, for occupational therapy, I had an hour-long session in a mock kitchen learning how to boil water and make noodles. Turning on the faucet was hard. As the pan filled with water, it became too heavy to hold. I asked myself, "How do I pour in the noodles? I could do this task at home before all this happened. Why is it so difficult now?" I thought, "*Press on, Helo; you have a family at home to feed.*" It was hard to lift the heavy pot of water, turn on the burner, open a box, and pour in the noodles. I forgot to turn the burner off, causing a potential fire hazard, so I didn't pass the cooking test. My husband and therapist stood by and watched. *I could not believe how hard this task was and how long it took me to accomplish it.* This was not the kind of cooking I enjoyed. One day, after repeated therapy sessions, I proved that I could safely cook simple things.

Chapter Six

CHANGES, CHANGES AND MORE CHANGES

Not everything that is faced can be changed,
but nothing can be changed
until it is faced.

— James Baldwin[1] —

Everything had changed and I was sick of it. Tired of relying on help, I just wanted to go home and have things return to normal, but life is in an ever-changing cycle. I knew that things would never be quite the same. I looked forward to going home and simply loving my family again.

While in rehabilitation sessions, I got to watch other patients carry out their own activities. It wasn't like going to a gym to work out. The skills we practiced in therapy seem simple to a healthy onlooker, but to a rehab patient, they're very challenging. Some patients were obviously struggling as much or more than I was. Others looked like they were on their last day, because they were doing extremely well. *They motivated me to keep pressing on.*

On the days my husband got to the hospital early, before lunch, I told him I was figuratively taking ten steps ahead in my recovery process because he gave my one hundred percent of his attention. Every time he arrived late, I told him that I felt like I was taking one hundred steps backward. *This was exasperating.* The nursing staff was wonderful, but I wasn't the only patient they had to attend to in the rehabilitation unit. Asking for their constant care wasn't an option outside of personal therapy sessions.

Sometimes, I called out for help from my room for what felt like an hour. "Help, can someone help me? Please, help!" And if I saw shadows of people walking by, or heard voices talking outside of my room, I yelled a little louder. *I think they were getting tired of my constant nagging. Understandably so.*

Unfortunately, I often forgot things due to short term memory loss. So what I thought was an hour of waiting, may have only been ten to fifteen minutes. I lost my call button frequently. Then a nurse came into my room, showed me the call button right by my side, hidden under the blanket. She patiently pointed out, "Helo, there is no reason for you to shout for help because you have a device right next to you to request assistance. Just hold onto it like this and push the button."

"I'm sorry," I mumbled.

"That's okay; just leave it on top on the blanket where you can see it."

That didn't help because I didn't remember where to leave it. Sometimes I'd just hold onto it and wonder why it was still in my hand. Over and over again, I'd forget, yell for help, learn about the call button remedy, then forget, yell, and learn again. My self care ability was very limited. My brain forgot things frequently, and having to wait for help resulted in impatience, making way for frustration, then agitation. *And I was embarrassed.*

When Rich was in the room I relied on him constantly. He helped to minimize my humiliation of having to ask others for help with basic tasks. When I requested simple things such as getting a blanket, a glass of water, assistance with eating or help going to the bathroom he attended to me right away. I never had to humble myself like this before surgery. I often thought, *"Are you kidding me, now I need help going to the bathroom?"* This shattered my dignity, but Rich's constant attention helped to restore it.

After weeks of walking in the hallways, it was time for me to venture out a little further. My physical therapist told me she was going to Starbucks right next to the hospital lobby. I remember asking her if she could get a coffee and a treat for me. She replied, "No, Helo. You need to go and get it yourself with my help." I told myself that I enjoyed Starbucks coffee and went for it. *It was a test of my endurance.* My husband and the physical therapist accompanied me. I walked down the hallway to the elevator, stepped in, went down several floors, and stepped out into the greeting center.

On this first visit to Starbucks during rehab, I felt a bit awkward and self-conscious because I looked and walked funny—and I was wearing that stunning blue hospital gown and robe—but I was happy to be out of my room. I ordered a Grande Decaf Vanilla Latte. I hadn't tasted anything that delicious in a long time. I sat down with my husband and physical therapist and enjoyed being out and watching the crowds. This adventure motivated me to want to get out again, but not too soon. After finishing my treat, I was exhausted. My husband took me back to my hospital room via a wheelchair. He tucked me into bed and I quickly fell asleep. In the days that followed, we ventured to Starbucks daily. It was great physical therapy.

On one of these trips, I was not allowed to use the elevator. I walked down the hallway to the top of a beautiful marble staircase with wide steps and glass sides. This was the most frightening walk down a set of stairs that I have ever experienced. My tilted double vision made the straight staircase look spiral instead. A black patch was put on one of my eyes, and that helped straighten the staircase for me. I was physically drained, but determined to get to Starbucks. My husband held on tight to my left arm as I held onto the banister with my right hand. It took me a long time to get down the stairs, one step at a time, with pauses of rest in-between. At the bottom was my reward: a Starbucks Grande Decaf Vanilla Latte and a Cake Pop. I sat again and rested, reminding myself that someday, I would be released from the hospital and enjoy Starbucks closer to home.

I knew I was getting better when part of my physical therapy consisted of getting into a van and going out to lunch. I could go anywhere. It was my choice and the hospital's treat. I had time to get dressed up if I wanted to. I felt exhausted and didn't want to go anywhere fancy for lunch, but the outing was not optional. I took a long nap to regain strength before my first required adventure off the hospital campus. I chose to go to Dick's Drive-in, a burger restaurant less than ten minutes from the hospital.

It took more than an hour and a half to get in the car, tolerate the ride, sit up, eat a burger, and then go back to my hospital room—and that was with the help of an occupational therapist and my husband. I thought, *"It's not supposed to take this much work to go out to lunch. How am I supposed to do this? Focus upon determination and tenacity, Helo."*

Later, I was happy to have ventured out.

My hospital stay was finally coming to a close. Rich went home to get some of my clothing—a nice change from hospital garb. One of my final assignments was learning to get dressed and undressed. This was easier to do after extended rest. At certain points during the day, I was simply too exhausted, so Rich helped me. Other times, he watched me and encouraged me to do it on my own. Sometimes I liked his approach; other times I didn't. He is a patient man.

One day, the room was very quiet. The nursing staff asked Rich to call for help if he needed it; otherwise, we were on our own. I had a private room. The curtain was drawn. The door was closed. Almost eight weeks had gone by.

"Rich, will you please snuggle with me?"

"I don't think that this is going to be easy, Helo. The hospital bed isn't big enough for the two of us."

"Please, I just need you to hold me. I can't remember the last time you did."

So he carefully got into my hospital bed, locked eyes with me, and we held each other tenderly. I was reminded of the previous time we were intimate—the night before I went in for surgery, only this time was so different. Last time I was several hours away from hospital admission—this time I was going home in a couple of days.

He gently stroked my head and said, "Helo, I love you. I can't wait for you to be back home. I've missed you for way too long."

I looked at the love of my life and flirted, "Rich make love to me right now."

It was a surprising request, and the smile on his face was the biggest one that I'd seen in quite a while.

"Are you sure?"

Smiling, I exaggerated, "Come and get it."

He grinned, "You, my beautiful wife, are quite the flirt."

I guess I didn't forget how to engage my husband.

Our intimate moment happened quickly. It was beyond beautiful because we got to treasure our marriage again. And we were reminded how much we missed each other. The next day, we repeated this encounter. Later, I asked for it again, but Rich told me to wait until we got home—we were leaving in just a few hours. Impatient, I did not want to wait, but I did anyway.

After eight weeks of hospitalization, I took off my hospital garb and eagerly got dressed with Rich's help. He opened the curtains and the sun shone through the window. I sat on the edge of the bed while he packed my belongings: clothing, pictures of my family, my Bible, cards, gifts of stuffed teddy bears, balloons, and a carved angel. We sat and listened to care instructions and signed off on a pile of paperwork. This was a lot more fun than signing the disclosures of risks before the surgery.

I was finally discharged!

My family and I were excited for me to go home, even though this journey would continue to affect us all. The discharge assessment documentation was lengthy. Among other things, it revealed:

Patient is able to negotiate level carpet around obstacles and people with occasional cues for posture and path. Patient needs cues to find her way in new environments. She is distractible. She can be easily re-directed. Her impaired attention negatively impacts her recall of presented information. She continues to have mild inconsistencies providing the exact date. She is not oriented to the month, year, exact date or her age. She is able to perform calculations involving five to six digits with seventy-five percent accuracy. She has difficulty performing equations involving subtractions. But during initial testing she performed one to two calculations with only fifty percent accuracy. She presents with double vision.

I exhausted easily and felt frail. The left side of my face was numb because of fifth cranial nerve damage. It felt like I visited the the dentist daily and received oral anesthesia but the numbness would not go away. A portion of my face felt deformed and sunken as a result of surgical incision of the temporalis muscle in order to gain access to my skull. And then there was constant double vision due to unavoidable disturbance of the nerves that move the eye.

I still had much to relearn and many challenges to face—but I was going home!

Packing up to go was complete. We said our "thank you's" and "good-bye's" to the Swedish Medical Center staff. Rich went to get our car, while I was wheeled out to the front of the hospital.

We had waited a long time for this day.

My husband drove up and I smiled from ear to ear. *I was dancing on the inside.* He and a nurse carefully helped me into the car. I looked back at the hospital, and whispered, "Thank you God for everything that You pulled me through."

During my entire hospital stay, I had over eighty thousand dollars of medication pumped into my body, contributing to the approach of one million dollars of medical care. Although overwhelmed, we were thankful for the phenomenal care I received. It felt incredible to be heading home.

As we rode together in the car it was as if I was seeing so much for the very first time again. Memories crowded my thoughts as I reminisced. The Seattle Space Needle reminded me of times together with my family. We drove by the University of Washington, where I'd met the love of my life, who was now driving me home. The arboretum was absolutely breathtaking. Every minute that went by was a cherished minute closer to *finally* returning home.

I'll never forget turning into our driveway after that lengthy hospital stay. The garage door opened. We drove in and I could not contain myself. *I was home!* I wanted to jump out of the car and exclaimed, *"Rich, hurry up!"* Instead, he gently lent a helping hand to get me out of the car, and held onto me tightly, as we carefully walked through the garage to the door of our kitchen. As I wobbled, he stayed by my side. He carefully helped me return home the same way that he had helped me leave months before. He is strong. I needed and need him to be that way.

I stood still, held tightly onto a railing, and anxiously waited while Rich opened the door for me. Everything looked brand-new. There were flowers on the counter, light shone through the windows, the sun glimmered outside, and the home was immaculate. The kids ran into the room, "Mom, you're home!"

"Yes, I am. I can't believe that I'm finally here. I wanted dad to drive faster on the way home, but he wisely ignored my request. Look at you! I missed you so much."

There were hugs all around. I reflected, "Time to marvel in the moment everybody, because God is amazing." After half an hour of beautiful reunion time, I was exhausted.

Rich walked me up to our room. A flower and note pad rested on the pillow. I read Rich's words of affection and said, "Thank you. I love you, too!" He helped me get dressed into pajamas, tucked me into bed, and between words of love, kissed my forehead. Further affection would have to wait.

My bed at home felt glorious, so I slept until the next day. The next morning, Rich helped me get dressed into sweats, brush my teeth, and make my way down the stairs. *It was not easy.* But I was finally home.

Chapter Seven

GOD IS AMAZING

Never be afraid to trust an unknown future to a known God.

— Corrie ten Boom —

While intubated in the ICU with a breathing tube, I communicated to my sister-in-law, motioning with a frail hand that I needed to write something. She handed me a pen and held onto a yellow pad of paper. This was the first time since surgery that I had initiated communication. I could've written anything, but what I wrote still moves me to this day. It took me five minutes with fragile hands to write three simple words, "God is amazing."

A year and a half later, I wrote:

GOD IS AMAZING

God is amazing.
His love is unmatchable,
And all I'll ever need.
I had nothing left to give,
Nothing to take along,
When I almost left behind those I love.
I never thought I'd walk this road behind or before me.
Frightened,
I cried out,
"God, I need You now."
Softly, I whispered as my strength was wearing thin,
And still He listened,
Because He hears our every prayer.

He never has, nor ever will leave my side.
He is my fortress.
He gave and gives me strength to find hope,
And press on.
In Him I found and find courage,
Not to quit.
He is all that I needed then and need now.
He heals fragile and broken hearts,
Removes discouragement, fear, and doubt.
He restores,
Takes away sin,
And makes me complete,
With perfect love,
The way that only He can.
One day I'll stand before Him,
And return to Heaven's door,
Suffering from affliction no more.
In awe, I'll fall to my knees in adoration,
Praising the only perfect love,
Because God is amazing.

— Helo

I'm often asked if I had a near-death experience. I reply, "I had a near-Heaven experience." It is a wonder that I am alive. One day, I'll stand at Heaven's door again. I imagine that I will fall to my knees when I see Him face to face. Or I will stand in awe, jump up and down, dance, sing "Hallelujah!" and lift up my hands in praise to the One who healed me in many ways. Or maybe I will be speechless before our God, who removes all pain and suffering when we enter His presence. Believe me, we are not there yet. His Kingdom delivers us and brings us to a beautiful place. "For you, Lord, have rescued my soul from death, my eyes from tears, my feet from stumbling, that I may walk before the Lord, in the land of the living."[1]

Suffering results not only from physical affliction, trauma encountered, and challenges endured, but also as a result of sin—from which none of us are immune. Yet God offers peace, grace, and forgiveness. St. Augustine once said, "God loves each of us as if there were only one of us." Now that is one amazing love. I now know that God will never leave my side through any challenge or difficult circumstance that I face. I now know what it means to find hope. I am continually moved by the truth of who God really is. He loves us, He is perfect, and knows how to address our suffering. "Behold, I will bring it health and healing; I will heal them and reveal to them the abundance of peace and truth."[2] God's healing can be physical. More importantly, God *alone* can restore us by reconciling us to Himself and making us spiritually whole.

When I first left the hospital, I was not independent but was happy to be home again. However, I was quickly reminded that I had a new normal that needed to be improved. In-home therapy was mandatory to direct my recovery. Little did I know that it would last twenty weeks.

A few days after my return home, my mother-in-law, Karin, came to stay with us for two weeks while I continued to recover. Karin had been a registered nurse in the ICU for many years. She was loving and tenderhearted, and continues to be. She kept us in daily prayer when I was in the hospital and had flown up from Florida to Seattle to stay with us.

Karin supported my efforts to be a more active wife and mom again. I am inspired by those who are as nurturing as she is. Incredible caretakers fully understand the necessity of balance between helping and honoring another's ability to struggle and grow through the healing process. It was hard for me to learn how to do everything over again, but I rose to the challenge with God by my side.

My mother-in-law facilitated in-home rehabilitation, ran errands, and took care of the boys. She wanted to see me get back on my feet again before she left. She helped me take steps towards recovery, even though we all knew it would be quite a while before I could walk any distance. Being back home was incredible, but in-home therapy wore me out.

Five days per week, I had three hours of in-home physical, speech, and occupational therapy. On the weekend, I continued with my husband's help. Karin scheduled appointments to make sure that I'd have rest time in between. I still slept up to nineteen hours a day.

I've always loved to listen and talk, but speech therapy? I looked at countless cards and was instructed to describe stacks of pictures to the therapist. At times I understood the pictures that I saw, but could not coordinate my thoughts and organize them into actual words. That collaboration of thoughts and speech didn't work for weeks. I saw a picture of an apple, a bird, or a flower and knew what it was, but I couldn't always make my mouth say it. My brain wasn't working the way it was supposed to, so my therapist gave me homework.

After learning how to describe pictures, I was taught how to read simple words…then harder ones. It felt like I had to start all over again, speaking like a child. I needed to be reminded that I was brave.

"Promise me you'll always remember: You're braver than you believe, and stronger than you seem, and smarter than you think."

— Christopher Robin to Winnie the Pooh[3]

In occupational therapy, I re-learned how to take care of the household. For example, I learned how to hold the handle of a broom and sweep again. Figuring out how to use a dust pan, to pick up the mess I had just swept into a pile, wasn't easy. I'd never liked cleaning dusty floors in the past, but in this case, I was resolved to master the skill again and enjoy it. And of course, I had to learn how to cook again. Determination to make my family meals, just like before, took hold. I started out with boxed macaroni and cheese with the help of my therapist, every step of the way—from opening the box to finally mixing in the powdered cheese. I repeatedly encountered what it means to be patient.

In physical therapy, my therapist helped me to walk first inside the house, to make sure I was steady on my feet. Then we walked outside, just down the driveway. She held onto my arm to prevent me from falling. Days later, we walked two houses down and back. We slowly added another house or two to our goal each week. My physical therapist was physically fit herself. I thought, "*She likely has never gone for a walk this slowly before.*" We walked rain or shine. I loved fresh air and found nature beautiful. I also discovered that even if we don't know where our journey is headed, we find hope when we take small steps of faith.

"Faith is taking the first step even when you don't see the whole staircase."

— Martin Luther King, Jr.

Although my emotions were normal, I experienced many post-surgery mood swings, and my crankiness did not dissipate overnight. Anyone who faces a near-death experience may revisit the trauma as intrusive memories make their unwelcomed appearance. I reminded myself that my journey had been a near-Heaven experience. I am alive today because God is amazing. *It was time to press forward.*

God is amazing, but I wasn't…at least I didn't feel amazing. I needed constant help at home, which was humbling. I slept a lot but didn't like sleeping time away. I got frustrated. I cried a lot. "God, stay with me please," I prayed. And He did. Nothing was easy. For instance, to make simple oatmeal for breakfast, I required my mother-in-law or children to help me get out the box of oatmeal, a bowl, and a spoon, and to heat it in the microwave. I wanted to do this all by myself. When I ate, I slobbered because I could open my mouth only about a half an inch and it took great effort to chew and swallow. I felt sloppy and embarrassed.

I couldn't walk up the stairs by myself. Going up required me to hold the railing on one side and someone's arm on the other side. Going down the stairs, I literally scooted on my bottom down one step at a time—

bump, bump, bump. I only did this twice a day because it was too hard to do and made me tired. Getting dressed required assistance, but over time, my husband and therapist insisted that I do it by myself. It took me way too long to get dressed. I chose shirts that didn't have buttons because they were easier to put on.

I had to use a special seat over the toilet and one in the shower. I couldn't read, so Rich handled all the bills. I wasn't steady on my feet, and my family worried that I might slip and fall. I couldn't drive, clean house, make meals, walk the treadmill, dance, or play the piano yet. There was a lot I couldn't do, but a lot I wanted to try. The one thing I missed the most was the ability to devote more time and attention to my family. I told myself, *"Stay on top of the therapy, Helo. Stay on top of it. One day you'll get to dote on your family again. Quality and quantity time will return."*

I had constant double vision for more than fifteen weeks. Everything seemed to be tilted. I saw one image in front of me and the exact image right next to it at an angle. I applied a sense of humor to this difficulty and as a result had two marvelous husbands in place of one and six incredible children instead of three—*or so I thought.*

I told my husband, "Number one gets to dote on and flirt with me and number two gets to clean house."

He responded, "I will choose to be husband number one over number two any day."

And so began official daily flirting and doting—and the enjoyment of an imaginary larger family. It was as if I saw the joys of my life, the craziness of my crooked vision, and began to laugh at myself as I discovered every new day was a blessing. I set goals each day: to make my own breakfast, to go up and down the stairs twice, and to complete therapy. Determination overcame discouragement, enabling me to succeed. I was highly self-motivated. I not only improved but also encouraged therapists and loved ones who wanted me to get better. They in turn encouraged me.

My in-home physical therapist told me, "Not all of my patients have the same determination to 'keep up the fight' that you have, Helo."

I replied, "I got my fortitude from my faith in God and my stubborn streak, mixed with determination, from my parents."

Stubbornness in this world has two opposite sides when it comes to how we think about God. We can choose to say that we do not need Him in attempt to face and accomplish everything on our own, or we can choose to be stubborn and exclaim that we will not do anything without Him. We then insist upon giving our battles or discouragement up to Him. That is when we get to see how amazing He is at loving and carrying us through adversity. I chose the latter form of stubbornness and in time found that it was, and is a beautiful choice. I do my best to not back down from loving God—because I know He loved me first.

By the end of the first two weeks of in-home therapy, I could walk down the stairs one step at a time, holding the railing with both hands. (Don't tell but sometimes I still scooted.) Over time, the things that I hadn't been able to do became doable. Rich played a pivotal role in this, as he started helping me less so I would learn to do more. Occasionally, he frustrated me by withholding help, but it was helpful in the long run. I now can accomplish many things by myself.

After I'd been home for two weeks, Dr. Tempest met with Rich and me to discuss my progress. Here is a portion of his notes:

Helo is ten weeks out from the excision of her left temporal microcystic meningioma. She continues to recover. Physically, she is independent in the house except coming downstairs, particularly if she is tired. Looking down at a staircase, for instance, she will see a spiral staircase rather than a straight one. She will fatique easily, and takes long naps during the day. She has a nice, full, smooth motion on her left side, but she notes it is still weaker than the right side. She is working with PT and OT daily and is partially independent in all self-care skills and mobility. She is doing her exercises daily for a minimum of three hours. She still has left facial numbness.

Cognitively, she still gets tired. She cannot read or see well. Even with glasses she has lost the ability to read. She is not yet doing any cleaning. Her mother-in-law is there this week. People are bringing in food. She does find, when she does some activities such as cleaning a room or emptying a wastebasket, that it takes her four times as long as it did before.

She has been out twice socially and was able to interact well without feeling overloaded, but she does get exhausted by the end of the day. However, this may be more of a mental fatigue. On physical examination, Helo walks without assistive devices. She walks well and smoothly, occasionally a bit haltingly. She has perhaps a bit more use of her arms than normal to maintain that balance, but nonetheless looks pretty good. Her language is clear and concise and she is continuing with speech therapy.

She outlines the numbness on her face. Emotionally, she feels that she is doing "Okay." She does not feel depressed but she does note things "build up" and she had an episode where she was really struggling. Cognitively, she is very likely to still have some impairments at high level function, information processing, short term memory, executive function, and multitasking. She needs to downplay these and focus more on the physical. We did talk about resumption of normal responsibilities as time goes on. Right now, she is focused primarily on her rehabilitation therapies, but I have encouraged her to start adding activities which she was responsible for in the past, like cooking, laundry, and some cleaning activities. We discussed her return to driving. It is not yet appropriate. I would like to get neuropsych testing done, but not yet. Helo is now ten weeks out from the excision of that large, but fortunately benign and completely excised tumor. Her brain and body will continue to recover. I suspect that it will be a matter of time.

Over time, with tenacity and determination—*I reached my new normal.*

Sometimes we face things that are beyond our comprehension and we become unsure about how to proceed. There were times when I privately came close to wanting to shake my fist into the face of God, but I never did because I recognized that this is what Satan wanted me to do in my discouragement. I persevered and kept trusting God.

I found hope, which encouraged my faith. This became a saving grace and fortitude. In Him, I know that I have a promise that I never have to face this or any other frightening journey alone. My neurosurgeon once told me that I was a fighter, but ultimately, God went before me in battle and instilled tenacity in me to find hope in Him.

Our struggles should not be downplayed because someone else is going through something "more" difficult. All afflictions are unique and affect us in various ways, both the one walking through the storm, and the one walking by their side. We are not to lose heart. It is all right to weep or feel as though we are at the end of our rope. *Having faith is sometimes hard.* But then we need to get back up again by the grace of God, put our trust in Him, and find hope in knowing that we don't ever have to be alone.

Returning home was a physical, intellectual, and emotional shock for me. I was happy to be back in our comfortable home and yet overwhelmed, mostly because I was amazed to be back. It took months before I could function as a capable mom and wife again, but I was well on my way. Rich returned to work full time, and I missed him every single day that he left. *I still do.* After Karin left, I continued therapy for almost five more months. I still couldn't make any meals, clean house, or run the household like before, so I humbly accepted help from friends and family.

It is easier for me to give than to receive. I love to help others rather than be served. For months, meals were brought to my home as arranged by a dear friend. Other people helped by taking our boys to various activities. Many people prayed and made themselves available to talk and listen. Many encouraged me and apparently, I listened and encouraged in return.

We all go through struggles that may parallel each other, but no two are exactly the same.

> *"Friendship is born at that moment when one person says to another: 'What! You too? I thought I was the only one.'"*
> — C. S. Lewis

I was once asked, "Helo, what was the hardest part of this journey?" I responded, "Patience." It is hard to be a "patient" patient when exhausted with having to learn to do so much over again. It is hard to say, "I think I can, I think I can!" but then have to stop because your body isn't cooperating or working in unison with the brain. I repeatedly tried hard and then shut down. It was hard to be patient then. Oftentimes, expecting to achieve something right away is not always the best way to get it. When patience matures, it will help us endure future challenges.

After months of in-home therapy, I experienced odd symptoms. Typically, in the middle of the afternoon, I attempted to get up and walk. I was obviously not paralyzed, but my legs felt like lead weights that did not want to move. I called my dad, asking him what this was. "It was a conversion reaction," he told me, meaning that the brain was not communicating effectively with the body. My brain had experienced a lot of trauma. My dad told me to talk out loud and instruct my legs to get up and walk. I needed to retrain my brain.

I thought, *"Talk to my legs? He must be kidding."* But he wasn't. So I followed his instruction. It did not work at first, and I sat down, frustrated.

The next day, I asked one of my kids to set my Bible on the table a few feet away from me. Remembering my dad's instructions, I stood up, looked down at my legs, and told them to walk. I took five steps, opened my Bible to a random verse, read it, turned around, walked away, and sat back down. Then I'd get back up again, walk back to my Bible to read another verse. This continued for several days. Finally, I had retrained a portion of my brain to cooperate with me. *At least when it came to walking.*

Playing the piano turned out to be one of my best therapies. When I tried to play, I could read most of the notes but couldn't make my fingers move and play them. I looked at Beethoven's Moonlight Sonata, a piece that I'd memorized decades ago. I thought, *"This ought to work. Look at the notes; read and play them, Helo. Simple, right?"* I understood what the notes were, remembered the melody, but could not transfer that information to my fingers. They weren't cooperating with my eyes. My brain was starting to annoy me.

Regardless of the annoyance factor, playing the piano turned out to be beautiful therapy. I started out with simple music, and in a determined manner, my brain eventually re-learned how to transfer the notes read by my eyes to my fingers. Finally, I got to tickle the keys, practiced my heart out, and refused to give up. I was convinced that one day I'd play the piano again, and eventually I did. I had never written a song before, but a year after returning home from my surgery, I wrote this simple song. I play it almost daily. My inspiration came from the Bible where it is written, "This is my comfort in my affliction, that your promise gives me life."[4]

I CAN SEE YOU, JESUS

Chorus

I can see you, Jesus,
I can feel You near.
And I know that You will never,
Never leave my side.

And I know that You will never,
Never leave my side.
Angels hold on tight,
Tell me everything will be all right.
Tell me if I stay or when I go,
God has my soul.

I can see you, Jesus,
I can feel You near.
And I know that You will never,
Never leave my side.

Verse 1
You are there when my soul and heart breaks,
And give me the hope that it takes.
You are there and give me your all,
Even when I lose faith and fall.

Please forgive my doubt filled with fear,
Crying out, hoping that You're still near.
Battles seem long and endless at times,
But your love is still strong and divine.

Verse 2
You are there and hold me so dear,
And You comfort my every single tear.
You are there to keep me brave and strong,
You will always be my heart song.

No more hold from affliction or fear,
'Cause your love's been made oh so clear.
I'm amazed by my Father above,
So I'll stand in awe of His love.

Verse 3
Unto You I give my whole heart,
And my life now has a new start.
In my faith, I stand on solid ground,
In You, my hope is always found.

You're the One that I choose to adore,
And then I want to know You even more.
Let this be my final hope and prayer,
That all will know that You're always there.

Twenty weeks of in-home therapy takes a long time—and I was getting a little antsy. Then one day I had a two-hour driving session with a certified disability driving evaluator. It was hard to believe that I was finally behind the wheel of a real car again instead of a make-believe metal one. I passed with flying colors, and the instructor legally vouched for my safe ability to operate a vehicle. All I needed now was for my neurosurgeon to determine whether I was at risk for seizures. After he concluded I wasn't, the Department of Licensing granted final approval for me to operate a vehicle—more than a year after surgery. I could walk, talk, dance, laugh, and drive. *God is amazing!*

Chapter Eight

RESILIENCE

The difference between a strong man and a weak one is that the former does not give up after a defeat.

— Woodrow Wilson —

Being resilient is accepting a new reality. It is time to recoil from the grip of adversity, not allow it to crush you, and choose to persevere instead. You can give up in defeat, adapt to simply survive, or press on with determination and be resilient. You can be stronger. *You can survive and soar.*

Your loved ones suffer when they see your pain. Mine suffered as they watched me. At times, life is hard. In those moments, look to God. Sometimes it might feel like He isn't there, but He always is. He loves us. He will never leave, nor abandon us. We need to understand that drawing near to Him, and asking Him to equip us with strength and determination, results in resiliency.

My husband and dad did their best to remain optimistic, but sometimes, feelings of helplessness consumed them. While I was in the ICU, my husband focused on the day that I would return home again, safe and sound. My dad practiced resilience by thinking forward to the start of my rehabilitation. At one point in the ICU—while my brother stood and watched—my dad told the lead neurosurgeon that he wanted to support my Achilles tendon at the back of my ankle with pillows. This would prevent the heel cord from shortening and thus protect my ability to walk so future rehabilitation would be easier. He was trying to think ahead.

My neurosurgeon looked directly at my dad and insisted, "I don't give a damn about your daughter's Achilles—I am just trying to keep her alive."

I was in a fragile state, and so was my family. If I could have, I would have reminded them of the strength of our Great Physician, whether I stayed here or went on the Heaven. "The Lord will strengthen him on his bed of illness; You will sustain him on his sickbed."[1]

From Greek mythology, an Achilles heel is a source of vulnerability. If the Achilles is attacked, defeat follows. In contrast, when we give our vulnerabilities to God, He goes before us in battle—He provides endurance and strength—and equips us to be brave.

> *"Even when I walk through the darkest valley, I will not be afraid, for You are close beside me. Your rod and your staff protect and comfort me."*
>
> — Psalm 23:4, NLT

My dad dealt with his helplessness by looking for ways to help me. If I came out of this, he wanted me to be ready for rehabilitation. His motto has always been "Things have a way of working out." But sometimes they don't—at least not the way we want them to. My dad just couldn't stand the thought of losing his daughter. There was nothing to do but pray. Nothing, and no one could guarantee that I would stay alive. That final outcome was ultimately up to God.

Our Achilles heels parallel our weaknesses. Sometimes we attempt to handle them on our own instead of letting go. God cares so much for us that He takes our weaknesses and makes us strong, and loves us in spite of them. Only God could fully comprehend the journey that my family went through. If possible, I would've reminded them to trust God: "Therefore let us draw near with confidence to the throne of grace, so that we may receive mercy and find grace to help in time of need."[2] We knew that "God loves us," but knowing this did not mean that our hearts would never ache. Whether I stayed alive or passed away, God would sustain my family. He would comfort those I left behind, and one day, I'd be reunited with those I love. This truth gave and gives me comfort.

Several months after surgery, I looked through my medical records for insurance purposes and accidentally came across a picture of the brain tumor still in my head. It was disturbing. I put the picture away within seconds and never looked at it again. My dad has a photo of the tumor completely removed and in a glass jar. As a physician and father, he is comforted by seeing concrete proof that the entire tumor was removed. For me, images of it are just painful.

One year after the surgery, I slowly began to investigate the details of the trauma that I had endured. I was amazed and simultaneously shocked to understand that being alive was a massive miracle. I did not fully comprehend the magnitude of what God had pulled me through, and I wanted to have a clearer understanding of what my family and I had endured. Then I remembered once again—*God imparts hope to the hopeless, rest to the restless, and courage to the discouraged. Time to accept the challenge and embrace resilience.*

I don't remember most of my hospital stay, which is a blessing. It's strange to have little memory of two months. Time was erased. It's odd to go into the hospital at the end of January and stay there through March wondering where all the time went. I was frustrated, physically and emotionally. I wanted to better understand what my family and I had gone through while I was hospitalized. But this could be a dangerous place to go.

A year and half after surgery, I explained my struggles to my brother, Henk over the phone.

Silence.

I asked, "Henk, are you still there?"

He tenderly responded, "Helo, I haven't told you this, because I wasn't sure when or if I ever should. But I took a picture of you in the ICU. One day, on my way to visit, I asked God for one-on-one time with my sister because I hadn't been alone with you yet. Every other time I visited, there was a doctor, nurse, or family member in the room with us. When I got to the room this time, there was no one else there. It hurt to see you on life support. I grasped your limp hands, closed my eyes for fifteen minutes, and envisioned our lives together. I got to see beautiful, fun, and difficult memories flash before my eyes. Terrified, I stood back and took a picture of you. I needed to preserve our precious time together."

My brother had shared this snapshot with no one for more than a year because it was "our private moment." He asked if I wanted to wait until Rich got home to look at the picture with him, but I was eager to see it, so my brother emailed it to me right away. I would look at it by myself.

The riveting picture shocked me. The scene was surreal, but it helped me to see what had happened. A tumor was taken out of my brain causing it to swell. I came close to dying multiple times. Shocking, I know, but that wasn't the entire story behind the photograph. The picture of me lying motionless gave rise to the miracle of healing that had occurred.

And now I was alive to look at it.

I called my dad and told him about the photograph. I emailed it to him, and he explained what we were looking at. It took him more than an hour to identify and describe every wire, tube, machine, and piece of equipment. More than forty wires and tubes had kept me alive.

Every single heartbeat was monitored while a respirator controlled my breathing. A central line, located above my collarbone, measured the intravenous pressure near my heart. Several lines administered medications, all on different time schedules. The total input of fluid was measured and monitored. The output of fluid was monitored through a catheter in my bladder. Sleeves around my legs were attached to pumps, squeezing my legs to prevent the formation of blood clots. A probe on my finger measured the oxygen saturation in my blood. There was also a suction portal, which the nurses used frequently to squeeze secretions out of my upper respiratory tract. Many probes were equipped with an alarm system, and all of the data was transmitted to the computer of an intensive care monitoring physician.

I later showed my husband the picture, and asked if this was really what I had looked like when I was on life support.

"I don't look like I am breathing."

He quietly said, "A machine did that for you, Helo. Your lungs inflated, your chest rose, and then stopped. The photo looks exactly like you did when your chest sank."

I sobbed. "I am so sorry that you and the kids had to see me this way." I stared at the picture for a long time.

Now I'm okay with looking at it. I carry a tattered copy around in my purse to remind me of the miracle God did, and I frequently share the picture with other people. They say things like, "You are beautiful, and this does not look like you," "Since you almost met God in Heaven, but He sent you back here, you must believe in Him even more," "You have an inspiring story to share," "You just put my day in perspective," "I thought I had things to complain about," "God has a purpose for you," and "Only God could have accomplished this miracle." Regarding my near-Heaven experience, I'm grateful for the journey. I wouldn't trade it for anything because of everything beautiful that I've learned as a result. *God is the triumphant One! I am not.*

At random times, I broke down emotionally. I had nightmares and woke up to intense feelings of fright and helplessness. Rich held me tightly to make me feel safe again. I experienced frightening flashbacks regarding diagnosis, surgery, and lengthy rehabilitation. Given the emotional and physical trauma I'd been through, it was natural to experience the acute symptoms of post traumatic stress disorder (PTSD). It was difficult to revisit these memories because they led to moments of depression and hopelessness. I felt angry, thinking that no one understood. But God did. I needed help to overcome acute PTSD but resisted the thought of seeing a therapist because I was exhausted and "doctored out."

I was thankful to be alive and wanted to display gratitude, not anger. God patiently gave me courage, but I still needed more help to prevent the PTSD from becoming chronic. I needed to learn to cope with the overwhelming fear and anxiety of almost dying so early in life. So I prayed.

One day, as I was feeling down, the phone rang. Whenever I answer a call from an unknown number and the caller mispronounces my name, I suspect that the caller is trying to sell me something. The phone rang, and the man on the other end of the phone asked, "Is 'Hee-low Matzelleeee' there?" I thought, "*Okay, what is the sales pitch?* I almost hung up on the caller, but I felt moved to listen. The caller, John, then informed me that he was with my healthcare provider, and he asked how my asthma was doing. I thought, "*He has no idea what I have been through if he's asking about my asthma!*"

And so I shared my story. After I told him about my surgery and recovery, John shared his story. He was a nurse who worked in psychiatry and had a brother who had just come back from Iraq, suffering from post-traumatic stress disorder. John himself had recently suffered a minor brain injury as a result of a bike accident. He told me that although our journeys were not exactly the same, he understood. He explained that it was completely normal for me to experience post-traumatic stress after coming so close to dying and having to relearn so much. He accepted my feelings of vulnerability, made me feel comfortable, gave me his number, and told me that I could call him any time.

God answers prayers in many different ways and showers us with His magnificent love so that, in turn, we can encourage and listen to others. I called and spoke to John for about an hour at least a dozen times. He supported me with wise counsel while sitting on my couch in the comfort of my own home. And as time went by, I learned how to better cope with the trauma that I had experienced. I explored my memories head on—safely. Over time it became easier, and PTSD was no longer a concern. *Resilience made itself known.*

* * *

One day, I sat at the computer, attempting to summarize my experience into a single page. The phone rang. I picked up, and on the other end was a representative from our lawn care company.

'Mike'[3] asked, "Why did you cancel your lawn treatment service?"

I quipped back, "A green lawn is not all that important to me."

He countered, "Green grass is important."

"Look Mike, I appreciate that you like green grass, but I'm in the middle of writing about a miracle that I've been through—and composing isn't an easy task. Besides, we chose yellow grass instead of green after facing an onslaught of medical bills. I need to go now."

"What miracle are you writing about?"

I shared my story.

Silence.

Mike stopped recording the phone call.

"Helo, you have no idea how much I needed to hear your story today. I've been suffering from depression for months. If a doctor told me that I had a tumor the size of a golf ball in my brain I'd likely shoot myself. If you can make it through this, I can make it through my depression. Your story is so captivating. It belongs on a movie screen."

Humbled, I then changed topic and we talked about what it means to be thankful to be alive. He told me to let him know when the book came out. I told him that I hadn't written a book before and had never thought that I'd have a reason to do so.

"You do now."

He thanked me for inspiring him.

I remarked, "Right back at you, you just inspired me."

The right person at the right time motivated me to keep writing in a moment when I wanted to quit.

Resilience followed by encouragement inspires us to press on when challenges surround us.

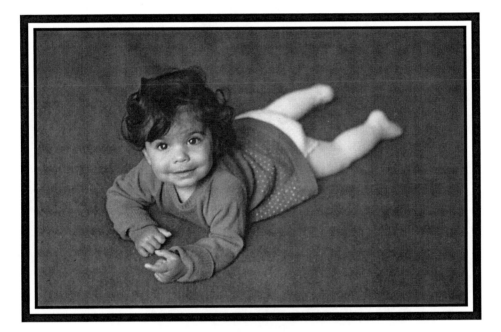

Helo at three months

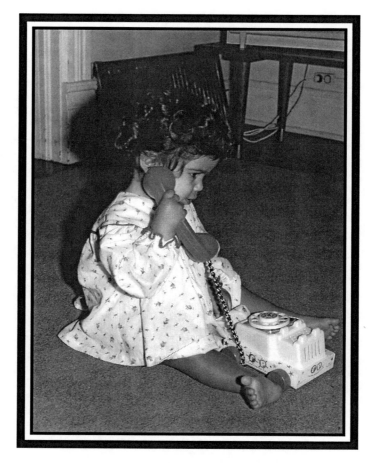

Helo making phone calls

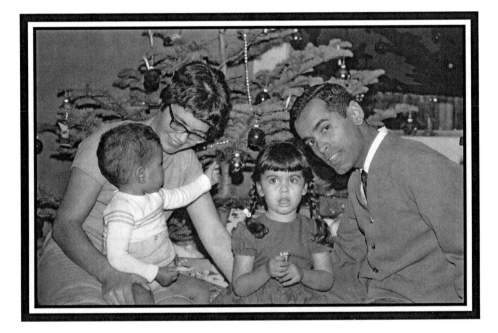

**A Dawson Family
Christmas
1968**

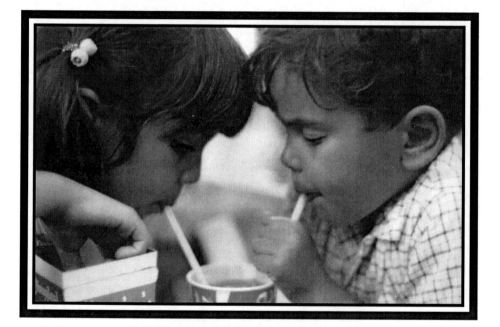

Sharing a soda with my brother

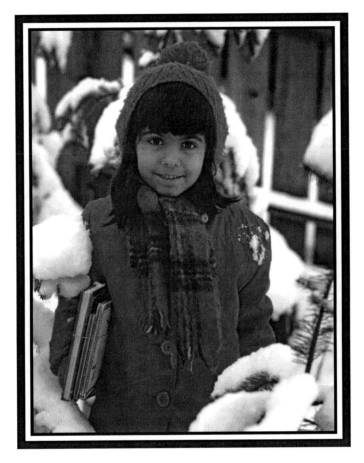

Back from the library

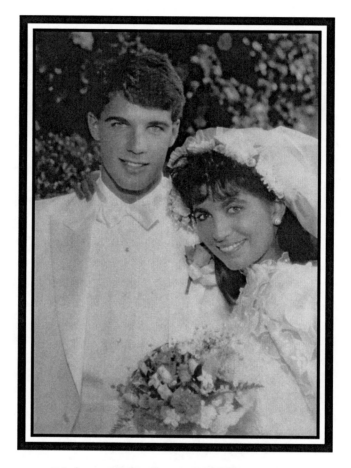

**Rich and Helo's Wedding Day
April 22, 1989**

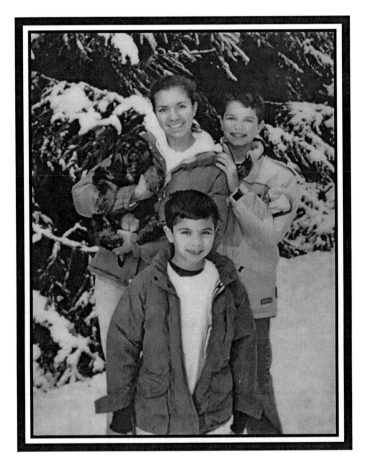

**Snow in Seattle
2004**

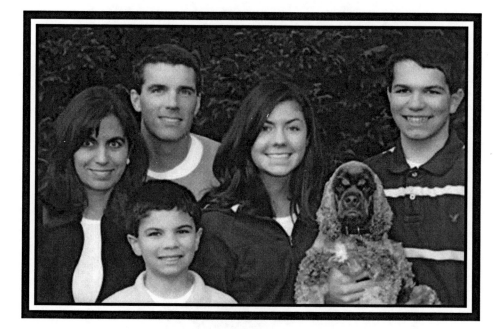

**Matzelle Christmas
2006**

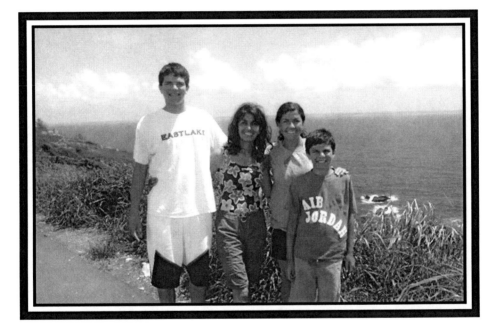

Helo and her three blessings

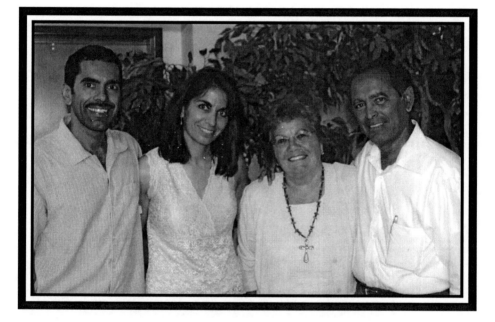

**Henk, Helo, Mom and Dad
A year before surgery**

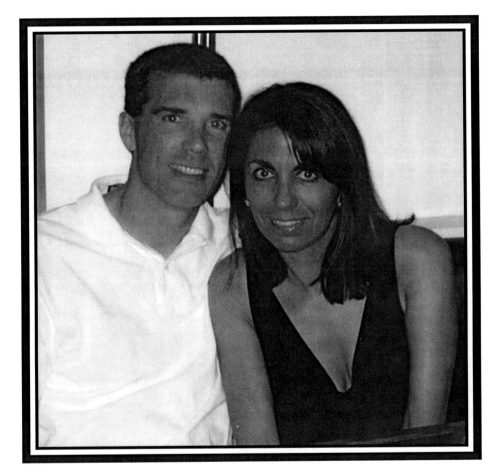

**Date Night
A few months before diagnosis**

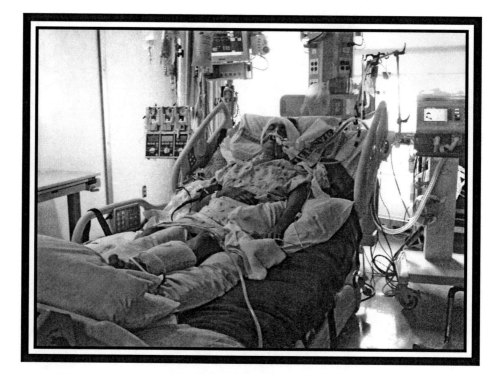

Helo in the ICU

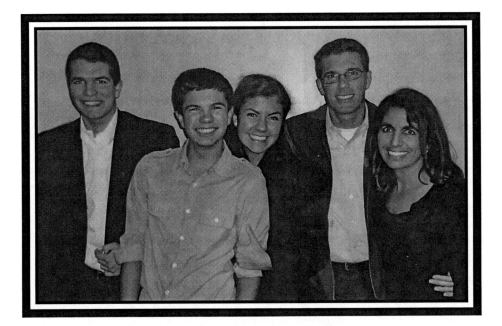

Matzelle Family Together
A year after surgery

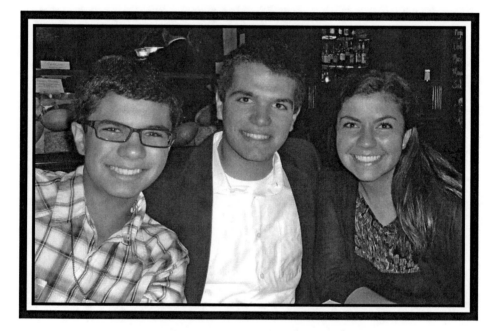

Austin(13), Jordan (16), Lauren (21)
Growing Up

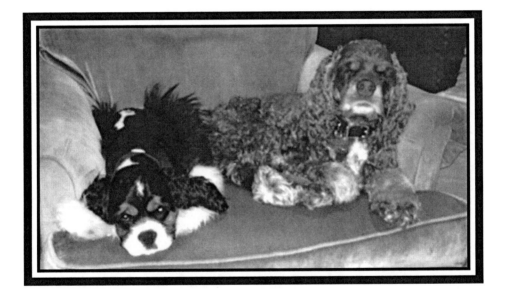

Buttons and Grace

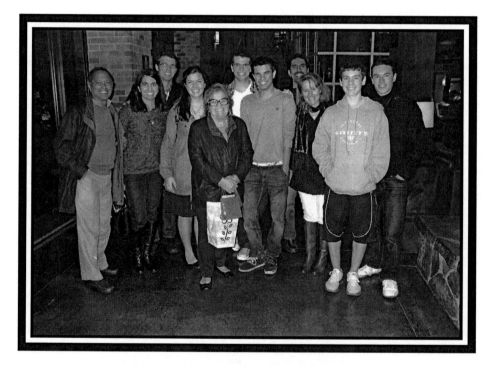

**Helo's family all together
Two years after surgery**

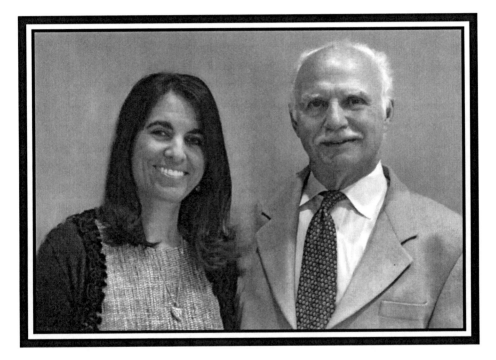

Helo with her earthly hero, Dr. James Raisis

Chapter Nine

TRANSPARENT DISABILITY

Move past the pity of disability and embrace the heart, mind, and soul of the person behind it.

— Helo —

I never asked for a handicapped parking placard to hang in the front window of my car, but one is there, because I am disabled. Sometimes, I look at it and ask God, "Why did this happen to me?" But He has a purpose for this journey. I now know what it means to find hope in uncertain and difficult circumstances, especially when I cannot see all of the reasons for the difficulties. I have chosen not to base my identity on the stigma associated with having a physical disability.

Sometimes it feels like I don't fit in or am not as strong, pretty, or successful as I'd like to be. I didn't deserve a miracle of this magnitude. I am not a hero. God is the hero in me. My faith is simpler and more complete than before because I now understand how amazing our God is. The Bible reminds us, "Now faith is the assurance of things hoped for, the conviction of things not seen."[1]

Once, while shopping at Costco, I parked in a handicapped stall. It was a busy day. The parking lot was full and there were fewer parking spots available than usual because of construction. As I opened the trunk, a frustrated woman yelled at me, "Get out of the wheelchair parking spot! Never park there again! You have no right to park there!"

I became teary because I wished at that moment that I did *not* have the right or need to park there. The ability to take a normal parking spot was something that I had taken for granted in the past. I told the woman that I recently had brain surgery, and she exclaimed that brain surgery had absolutely nothing to do with the ability to walk. Well, she was clueless. Sometimes people in their frustration say the meanest, stupidest things. I've even had people ask, "When is the tumor coming back?" They don't intend to hurt me, but they would do better to be silent.

When someone mistreats you, look at it as a moment to grow in grace. Keep your focus on God rather than on retaliating or saying something mean back. Satan takes part by discouraging us in an attempt to bring us down. I not only tell him to get behind me but also tell him to keep his mouth shut. Then I move forward by setting my mind back on God and asking Him to carry me.

Months later, I went to Safeway to make a quick grocery stop. My boys had eaten a key ingredient for dinner that evening. Prior to surgery, I would have given my boys a lecture on how they are not supposed to eat the ingredients before the meal is ready. They had obviously forgotten the food-consumption rules in our home. After surgery, I forgot things quite often, too. I didn't feel that the symptom of short-term memory loss was contagious except when I dealt with my teenagers. On this day, I had chosen to smile instead of lecturing them. I was thankful that I had the ability to go shopping, make a meal, and enjoy my family's company.

An older man who worked at the Safeway led me out to my car and pushed my cart through the pouring rain. He questioned, "I hope you don't mind my asking you this, but why do you have a wheelchair tag in your car? You look just fine." In the past, if someone I didn't know had talked to me in a parking lot in the rain, I would not have wanted to get soaking wet and discuss personal matters.

But God had pulled me through something that changed me, so we stood in Seattle's notorious rain. I told the man my name and shared the journey that I had been through, including what God had done to restore me. I hadn't asked for his name, because I didn't need to. He looked at me and explained the struggle that he and his wife were going through financially. They had moved to be closer to their children, but unfortunately their children moved away. His wife was struggling emotionally.

He explained, "I am now in my seventies. I was raised Pentecostal but never have thought of myself as being good enough for God. But your story has inspired me, Helo."

I was completely soaked in the rain and was reminded that God showers His love over us. I looked at this man and said, "'James,'[2] you do not need to be good enough for God, none of us can be."

Shocked, he looked back at me and remarked, "Whoa, Helo, you are good at this. How on earth did you know my name?"

I smiled, and so did he after I countered, "Because you are wearing a name tag."

He laughed and snickered, "Uh-oh, guess I got absorbed in our conversation."

A moment of silence went by in the rain, and then I revealed, "Anyway, James, God does not need a name tag for you. He knows your heart, mind, soul, mistakes, regrets, and hopes. He made you, and He loves you."

James told me he needed to start going to church again, but he might move away soon and didn't want to start attending one only to stop and attend a different one later. I told him that he didn't need to wait until Sunday to spend time with God.

Moments of silence went by.

James asked, "Are you a pastor?"

"No, I'm neither a pastor, nor theologian. I'm just a blessed and cherished child of God, and so are you."

James replied, "I now know that I need to spend more time with God. I haven't done that for a long time."

I said, "God would love that, and you will find out how much He adores you."

After a few moments, James commented, "I am going to ask my wife to spend time with God. She needs Him, too."

I thought, "*We all do.*" James and I stood in the Safeway parking lot, soaking wet. He thanked me for listening, and I thanked him back, then got in my car and drove home. This had been an inspiring moment for both of us.

*   *   *

I now pray for everyone whom I see in a wheelchair. One morning was a little different because I did more than just pray. It was before eight a.m., and I had to take my son to the orthodontist to replace a retainer that our delightful puppy, Buttons, had chewed up. She has expensive taste in chew-toys and is too cute to get into serious trouble. I brought our dogs, Grace and Buttons, with us to the orthodontist so everyone else could sleep in.

I parked in a handicapped spot, and my son Jordan went into the orthodontist's office. Moments later, I noticed a man lowering the wheelchair ramp of his van. He carefully wheeled a young girl into the vehicle. The ramp made a lot of noise as it moved back into its place. The man made sure that the girl was securely locked in. Her wheelchair was loaded with equipment. Their situation looked intense.

I grabbed Buttons, got out of the car, and said, "Hi, my name is Helo. I don't mean to interrupt you, but would you like to see my puppy, Buttons?" Normally, I would not have done this. Buttons was still young and typically barked at strangers. She didn't like large new objects and would playfully growl and then bark at them. This time she didn't.

The young girl was obviously disabled. Her arms and legs could not move easily, and she was quite frail. Her speech was impaired, but she could talk. The wheelchair was heavily equipped with electrical devices. Buttons ignored all of this, jumped onto the tray of the wheelchair, and licked the girl. I hadn't seen Buttons behave that way before. The girl and her father lit up.

I told the girl that she was very good with animals and that maybe she would grow up to become a veterinarian. She said that she loved dogs but did not want to go to school for long enough to become a vet. When she had been in the hospital after neck and back surgery, she told me that she'd had a dog visit her every day. She'd convinced the owner of the dog to allow his companion on her bed, against regulations. It was the best medicine she had ever received. She insisted it was better than drugs, shots, tubes, wires, or doctor visits. I told her about the visits that I'd had with a dog in the hospital. I agreed that they were great medicine. I told her that good dogs love protectively and happily but don't evaluate medical conditions. It was nice to get a short break from medical evaluations. She agreed.

I told her that she had a twinkle in her eye, and she pointed up and exclaimed, "It comes from God." She confided that it was hard to be disabled, and that people left her out of things because they did not like to include her. "That really hurts," she told me. She loved music and wanted to learn how to play the piano, but her fingers were not strong enough. She also told me, "People can be mean." She had her fifteenth birthday coming up, and one boy had told her that she could invite him to her party, but shouldn't expect him to want to spend any time with her. She told me that if people don't have anything nice to say, they should just keep their mouths shut. I told her to be sure to celebrate her birthday and that God had made her beautiful.

I then shared with her how people were sometimes mean to me and asked me when the tumor was coming back. I shared the story of how someone had gotten really mad at me for parking in a wheelchair spot at Costco, even after I had explained what had happened to my brain. The girl interjected, "Brains are important. I don't know what I would do without mine. I can't use it the way others can. I have to be slow and do one thing at a time. Right now, I am talking to you. After that I am going to focus on Buttons. Wow, she is so cute."

I was about to leave, but her dad looked at me as if to say, "Keep going, Helo. Keep going." The girl told me that she felt trapped inside her body and wanted to be normal like everyone else. People sometimes ostracized, ignored, or made fun of her. I could tell by the look on his face that this hurt her father deeply. The three of us agreed that people often don't know what to do when they see someone who is disabled. But today, the dad told me, someone had known what to do. He couldn't thank me enough for stopping to talk and share Buttons with his daughter because this sort of thing rarely happened.

While Buttons and I were visiting, my other cocker spaniel barked incessantly. The girl asked me, "Who's in your car?" I told her that it was Grace and that sometimes, at home, Grace upsets me and when I exclaim, "Grace!" my kids quip back, "And peace be with you, Mom." The dad smiled, and the girl laughed, saying, "I think Grace wants to be with me and Buttons. She has something to say." Grace stayed in the car. Buttons, on the other hand, was having a grand time. She accidentally and then intentionally pushed buttons on the wheelchair; it lit up and beeped. She repeated this over and over again. The girl burst into heartfelt laughter. I laughed on the inside, and the dad smiled.

When it was time for me to go, I gently took Buttons away. She jumped out of my arms and back onto the wheelchair tray as if to say, "I am not leaving." The girl's dad insisted, "We need to take you to school now, dear." She responded, "But Dad, I don't want to go to school. I want to stay here with Buttons and Helo."

I told her she had a bright light inside of her and that God was going to take her places. One day, perhaps she would go to the hospital with a dog and help others because she was very good at it, I suggested. She smiled with that twinkle in her eye. By that time, her dad had pulled up the ramp. He shut the door, looked at me, and smiled. "Thank you, Helo. You have no idea how much you just brightened our morning." I said, "Right back at you." He walked away to get into the van, raised his arms, pulled them back down, and exclaimed, "Yes!"

I paused and rejoiced, "Yes, thank you, God, for all that you do!"

I had listened to this tenderhearted girl who loved God even though she was teased by onlookers and "friends." We all face different and diffi-cult challenges. Many people have told me that my journey is unbeliev-able and that theirs pales in comparison. To this I say, all of us have, or will face different challenges. But the point is that we can face our battles by God's grace. When we humbly allow God to equip us for His glory, we will be blessed with opportunities to encourage others. Then encouragement often comes right back at us, sometimes tenfold. That is a blessing, and Jesus taught us to encourage and bring hope to others:

> *Blessed are the poor in spirit,*
> *for theirs is the kingdom of Heaven.*
> *Blessed are those who mourn,*
> *for they will be comforted.*
> *Blessed are the meek,*
> *for they will inherit the earth.*
> *Blessed are those who hunger and thirst for righteousness,*
> *for they will be filled.*
> *Blessed are the merciful,*
> *for they will be shown mercy.*
> *Blessed are the pure in heart,*
> *for they will see God.*
> *Blessed are the peacemakers,*
> *for they will be called children of God.*
> *Blessed are those who are persecuted because of righteousness,*
> *for theirs is the kingdom of Heaven.*
> *Blessed are you when people insult you, persecute you and*
> *falsely say all kinds of evil against you because of me. Rejoice*
> *and be glad, because great is your reward in Heaven, for in the*
> *same way they persecuted the prophets who were before you.*
> — Matthew 5:3–12

Many of us have disabilities, some more visible than others. I have had significant trauma to my brain—but hardly anyone can tell by just looking at me. I have a friend whose son has brain damage. God continually gives my friend strength to take care of her son, and she now helps others in similar situations. Those who suffer, but humbly seek out God's purpose for allowing difficulty, are blessed. I never asked for a wheelchair tag to be mounted in my window, but God has obviously used it for me to minister to others. I am not backing down from sharing what He has pulled me through and all that I've learned in the process.

My face is now permanently numb on the left side so I don't respond to kisses on my left anymore, because I can't feel them. I didn't want my husband to think that I was ignoring his affection if he kissed me on the wrong side, so one day I used a marker to draw a heart on the healthy side of my face. This reminded my husband which cheek to kiss.

I am blessed that I don't have muscular damage on the left side of my face, because when I smile, no one can tell that I cannot feel most of my expression. I do have a permanent indentation next to my left eye because of muscular atrophy of the temporalis muscle. Since a portion of my face feels constantly numb, and the top of my left skull feels tight—sometimes this makes me feel deformed.

Today, I tire very easily and "hit the wall" frequently. Accomplishing simple tasks still takes me three to four times longer then it used to. I lost more than half of the hearing in my right ear; the cause is unknown. There is no surgery or hearing aid that can fix it, and it will never come back, but care is taken to preserve what little is left. There are silver linings: I no longer hear my husband snore when I sleep on my good ear and don't need to tell him to stop making a racket. When I talk to people on the phone on my right side, their voices sound elevated, making them sound like Alvin the Chipmunk. This is funny at times; at other times, it's frustrating. God gives us a sense of humor to cope with challenges or difficulties. Laughter can be both necessary and therapeutic.

I have a new normal now. I cannot do all of the tasks that I used to, but I wouldn't trade my blessings, found as a result of this trial, for anything. I am now more transparent in communicating what God wants me to share as a result of becoming transparently disabled.

Chapter Ten

HE ANSWERS PRAYER

Rejoice in hope, be patient in tribulation, be constant in prayer.

— Romans 12:12 —

I have moments when my hope diminishes and doubt sets in. Doubting is equal to thinking that God cannot address our requests perfectly—it's also a symptom of lack of trust. So, when doubt sets in, I reach out to God in prayer. I simply cry out to Him and wait. Sometimes He answers right away, and sometimes it takes a long time. That long wait in itself is His answer: He is asking me to be still and patient. It's not like I can make a request known to God, and He answers right away, "Here you go, Helo." In His wisdom, He does not work like that.

At other times, I think that I can fix my situation on my own. This is when I am fighting hard to follow my own agenda instead of carrying my burdens to God in prayer. However, time and time again, this approach has failed. Prayer replaces discouragement. Talking to God quietly or out loud is extraordinary and a privilege. He is forever faithful. He knows us better than anyone else and will meet us wherever we are. He is our comfort, our shield, and refuge. By spending time with Him, we get to know Him and acknowledge who has authority over our lives. He is one amazing love. Prayer is an opportunity to talk to Him, ask Him questions, thank, and praise Him. "Give thanks to the Lord, for He is good; His love endures forever."[1]

Prayer is not complicated. It is simple. It can take place at any time, anywhere. Prayers can last for hours—or be short and sweet. They can also be straight to the point like, "God help me!" His answers to our prayers might come right away or take a long time. In the process, we get to learn how to be patient, or learn what it means to be surprised! Either way, we can be brought to a place of awe. "Call to me and I will answer you and tell you great and unsearchable things you do not know."[2] I've learned that He listens to every single request. He never stops.

Several months after returning home, I walked into a grocery store and started to cry, not caring if anyone saw me. I was quietly asking God if I would grow old enough to meet my grandchildren. I watched the preoccupied people in the store busy with their day. I pulled a bag of tortilla chips from the shelf and physically bumped into an elderly woman.

She fixed her eyes upon me and asked, "Can I pray for you?"

People whom I had never met have prayed for me, but this was the first time in my life that I had bumped into a complete stranger who immediately asked me if I needed prayer.

At first I told her, "No, thank you."

But she repeated, "Can I pray for you, please?" She did not give me a chance to respond and told her husband to go get yogurt.

I looked at her cart and commented, "Your cart is full of yogurt. Why on earth would you want more?"

She grinned, saying, "Yogurt is at the other end of the store, my dear. If I send my husband to the yogurt section, I will get to spend more time with you."

Her husband smiled, and asked, "Got ministering to do?" He graciously left to "get yogurt." What he really did was wander the store aimlessly and give his beloved wife time with me. I later learned that the woman's name was Faith. She held my shaking hands, looked directly into my tearing eyes, and asked me to share what was going on.

I shared the story of my brain tumor that rested over my carotid artery and what had followed. Then I explained my fear of not growing old enough to meet my grandchildren. It was consuming me.

This is when I learned that our prayers are heard and answered when we completely relinquish fear, don't attempt to outline the answers we desire, and trust in Him. Our prayers will be addressed and answered by Him in His perfect timing and sometimes in amazing ways that will delight us.

Faith said, "I am seventy-two years old. I have fourteen grandchildren. Thirty-five years ago, I had a tumor on my carotid artery. Granted, my tumor was not in my brain; it was in my neck. But you see, medicine thirty-five years ago was much different than it is today. The tumor was removed, but the surgery put me at risk, and the recovery was scary, too. So, when I tell you that I understand your fear of potentially not growing old enough to meet your grandchildren, I mean it." She then prayed over me.

God put this woman, Faith, in front of me just at the right time. I could not have ever come up with a better answer to prayer. Shortly after expressing to God my anxiety of not growing old enough to meet my grandchildren, while walking through a grocery store, He introduced me to someone who completely understood my apprehension and quenched my fear of *tomorrow* when I needed it the most. Comfort set in. My fear left me, and I saw that God is our Protector. My encounter with Faith doesn't necessarily mean that I will be guaranteed to live long enough to meet my grandchildren—that is ultimately up to God. But meeting Faith answered my prayer on that day. I remembered that we are not to worry about tomorrow because today has enough worries of its own.[3]

He sustains us and answers prayers in incomprehensible ways: "Then they cried to the Lord in their trouble, and He brought them out of their distresses. He caused the storm to be still, so that the waves of the sea were hushed. Then they were glad because they were quiet, so He guided them to their desired haven."[4]

God's answers to prayers are endless, and often He answers them in unexpected ways. One day, a year and a half after my surgery, my family and I went to a beautiful lakefront park on a sunny day. I remember sitting on the lakeshore talking with my daughter, Lauren. Being able to do so meant a lot to both of us. She had just graduated from an undergraduate university and was wait-listed for law school. She had been nannying throughout the summer and didn't know what to do next. She got up to go swim in the lake with her brothers and dad. I thanked God for her and then began to pray for her future. While she was swimming her cell phone rang, but I didn't pick up the phone. Someone from the University of Washington School of Law had called and requested a return phone call. We later learned it was the Director of Admissions.

My husband and I held back premature celebration. We thought that there could only be one reason that she had been called. Over the weekend, I searched our family closets for the university's colors. We had plenty, given that we are Husky fans. I planned for all of us to wear something nostalgic in honor of her future Alma Mater and to celebrate her acceptance.

Monday arrived, and Lauren called the university. After she'd been on the phone for what seemed like a long time—about thirty minutes—I finally broke down and listened in. The only part of the conversation that I heard was when Lauren said that she'd be honored to accept an offer of admission. I jumped up and down at the bottom of the stairs! *"Thank you, Jesus! My daughter is going to become a lawyer! And she is going to be a fantastic one. God, you are amazing."*

Lauren came down to share the good news, and I was thrilled for her. I almost cried because I'd come so close to losing the chance to hear her great news, but that, in and of itself, reminded me of how incredible God is and how magnificent His answers to prayer are.

God already knows our prayers in advance. If we stop and reflect on this, we will stand in awe of Him. He has the power of foresight and hindsight. We have the gift of hindsight alone, and we shouldn't bother to worry about tomorrow. "Therefore do not worry about tomorrow, for tomorrow will worry about itself. Each day has enough trouble of its own."[5]

At times, we cry out and wonder how He will answer our prayers. I've learned that He alone has the ability to answer our solemn requests in beautiful and unpredictable ways. At times, we pray and wonder why He hasn't answered yet. Remember, this can be an answer in itself, as He calls us to be still. Only He knows what is best for us. "I love the Lord, for He heard my voice; He heard my cry for mercy. Because He turned his ear to me, I will call on Him as long as I live."[6]

My family often had to combat anguish with prayer, especially when I was in the ICU. Through the entire process, they offered prayers of thanksgiving and requests for healing. My family prayed earnestly, motivated by their love for me. God enabled them to press on as they waited to get their Helo back.

When I finally came home, people sometimes "wished me luck" or kept their fingers crossed for me. This sort of encouragement, although thoughtful, was not enough for me. I needed to go deeper than that. So I immersed myself in prayer and discovered its comfort and power.

Now I pray for others boldly. I understand that I don't have to know absolutely everything about their stories to pray effectively. Our Father knows every last detail and the Holy Spirit helps us pray:

> *Also the Spirit helps us with our weakness. We do not know how to pray as we should. But the Spirit himself speaks to God for us, even begs God for us with deep feeling that words cannot explain. God can see what is in people's hearts. And He knows what is in the mind of the Spirit, because the Spirit speaks to God for His people in the way God wants. We know that in everything God works for the good of those who love Him.*
> — Romans 8:26–28, NCV

Since my surgery, people have disclosed a lot of private struggles to me. Perhaps this is because I keep them confidential. It is humbling to be trusted like that. I hold onto the conviction that God can handle it all—perfectly. And frankly, knowing who the Master is makes it easier to listen to others' heartfelt challenges—then I don't have to take their troubles upon my own shoulders. Instead I relinquish troubles to the One I trust. He alone can handle everything with grace and fortitude. *That's assurance at its best.*

Sometimes I feel like I've got enough on my plate—but I love to pray for others. Many of my closest friends have gone through difficult journeys: Cancer. Loss of a loved one. Anxiety. Financial stress. Infertility. Divorce. Depression. Loneliness. And more.

After raw pain is disclosed, I tell them that I'm not going to bring it up when we talk, not because I don't care—but because I do. I tell them to bring it up when they want to; I won't ask a lot of questions, if any. Inquisition sometimes unravels us and hurts, especially when we are not prepared for it. And besides, I'm not a qualified counselor. But I know how to pray.

Dear friend, "You can bring it up with God any time. When we talk, I want to be a safe friend. I can pray for you without knowing every last detail, because God already knows them all." This allows for much needed moments of normalcy during trials. It's okay not to be okay; sometimes we just need moments to breathe and the quiet comfort of a friend. Sometimes we need to set our burdens aside and focus on all that we have to be thankful for. In Him, our sustenance is found. I've learned, over and over again, that what we need the most is one-on-one time with God.

I pray when I get up in the morning, when I go for a walk, when I sit down for a meal, when I feel thankful and joyful, when afraid, when a friend asks me to, when my family needs me, if I've had a bad dream, before and during a doctor's appointment, when in traffic, when my husband travels, when around family, when I hear upsetting news, when I am at church, and while running errands. I offer up prayers of thanksgiving every time I stop and reflect upon my Savior. I have learned to "Pray without ceasing."[7]

I pray with thanksgiving and praise to our amazing Father, who loves me abundantly.

I pray for my husband, and for protection over our marriage, thanking God for giving Rich to me.

I pray for my children, asking that they will continually learn how to stand steadfast in their faith.

I pray for my parents and thank God for giving them to me.

I pray for my extended family and friends, resting in the knowledge that God already knows where they need His grace.

I pray for leaders.

I pray for peace in this world.

I pray for everyone who has a wheelchair tag in their car.

I pray for those I see in a doctor's waiting room.

I pray every time I see an emergency vehicle with lights flashing.

I pray for pregnant women, hoping for safe deliveries and healthy children.

I pray for people driving around me. (I do this without closing my eyes, in case you are wondering.)

I pray for the nearly seven hundred thousand people in the United States, as well as for others around the world living with brain tumors today. I pray for a cure, so that one day, this affliction will vanish.

I pray for people with challenging diagnoses.

Whenever I see a homeless person, I pray over him or her for shelter, food, and restoration.

Whenever I see a school bus, I pray for the children on board, their families, and the driver.

I pray for protection over my thoughts when I face moments of frustration, fear, weakness, or anger.

I pray for those facing depression.

I pray for those who do not yet know Jesus.

I pray for those who do know Him.

I pray for those afflicted and ask that they will find strength, hope, and faith.

I offer up prayers of thanksgiving each day, when I see my husband and children and realize how enormously blessed I am.

I offer up prayers of gratitude when I wake up in the morning because I am alive.

I pray to God asking Him to keep me humble.

I pray to ask God how He wants me to live.

I thank God for all that He gave and gives.

Through prayer, we are renewed. We receive the joy of walking with the Author and Perfecter of our faith. Prayer is not about putting on a Christian facade, acting "holier than thou," or pretending that we are morally perfect. *None of us can be.* At times we attempt to have conversations with God on our terms, not His; mistakenly thinking we can hide the broken parts of ourselves from Him. *Dear one, He sees it all. Always.* When we finally understand this, we will recognize that He knows us better than anyone else. Then we discover the hope of endurance by praying to the One who loves us.

Prayer is about fixing our eyes humbly upon Christ: "...Let us also lay aside every encumbrance and the sin which so easily entangles us, and let us run with endurance the race that is set before us, fixing our eyes on Jesus, the Author and Perfecter of faith, who for the joy set before Him endured the cross, despising the shame, and has sat down at the right hand of the throne of God."[8] As a result of fixing our eyes on Jesus, we learn how much he loves us, and we can turn around and genuinely love others. I love this Prayer of St. Francis, keep it hanging on my kitchen wall, and reflect on it often:

Lord, make me an instrument of Your peace.
Where there is hatred, let me sow love;
Where there is injury, pardon;
Where there is doubt, faith;
Where there is despair, hope;
Where there is darkness, light;
And where there is sadness, joy.
Oh, Divine Master, grant that I may not so much seek to be
consoled as to console;
To be understood as to understand;
To be loved as to love;
For it is in giving that we receive;
It is in pardoning that we are pardoned;
And it is in dying that we are born to eternal life.

To that I say, "Amen," and I stand in awe of how He answers prayer.

Chapter Eleven

NO COMPLAINING

If you don't like something, change it. If you can't change it,
change your attitude. Don't complain.

— Maya Angelou —

Complaining is contagious, but so is the opposite, including appreciation and gratitude. Negative words bring ourselves and others down. Positive words lift ourselves and others up. Simply choosing to be thankful makes every day beautiful and eliminates room for complaints. "In everything give thanks: for this is the will of God in Christ Jesus concerning you."[1] It is easy to grumble about struggles, but then we lose sight of what God is doing with our adversities to make us strong.

When I returned home after almost taking my final breath, I was overwhelmed and humbled by God's miracle. This journey shattered me to the core. It also grew me in big ways. Priorities and perspectives changed. Keeping the house immaculate and running the household mattered to me, but not as much as it had before. Besides, I am thankful for the mess makers, including myself.

I now have a new normal. Fatigue happens. Tasks take a lot longer than they used to. I don't have the ability to hear well and feel that I'm constantly repeating myself. I forget things and sometimes don't remember whether I've asked my husband or children to do something. My children sometimes use this to their advantage—oftentimes in a delightful way. I have found that my memory issues can cloud every day occurrences, but unique events are not forgotten.

Following my surgery, physical and emotional challenges competed with my determination to conquer discouragement. I desperately wanted to be better and whole again—for myself and for my family. When I couldn't master a challenge, I'd fall down in disappointment and complain, and if I took small steps forward, a thread of hope was woven and complaining melted away.

Given a second chance at life, I mistakenly thought that I needed to be perfect, never complain, and appreciate everything, as if I had to earn God's mercy. My need to be perfect affected my closest relationships. I wanted to be an "awe-inspiring" wife, mother, daughter, sister, and friend. All interactions were supposed to be open, without up and downs, and unconditionally loving...or so I thought. I was afraid that one day too soon, goodbyes would be repeated, only this time for good. If I ever put my family or friends through an ordeal like this one again, I did not want any of us to harbor regrets, or to look back and say, "I wish I could have said 'such-and-such' to you before you left." I thought every day was supposed to be flawless in case it was our last. I told myself, *"Always be patient and slow to anger. Unceasingly listen, never argue, maintain a sense of humor, and never be offensive. Encourage those around you and support every endeavor, never discourage, and love unconditionally. Never hold love back. And never, ever complain. Always have faith. Cherish and adore your husband, children, family, and friends. Always."*

I haven't completely succeeded at this and never will. It was unreasonable to think that I could. Then I'd complain about my inability to be a perfect mom, wife, daughter, sister, and friend. This thought pattern was wrong. My family and friends are ultimately cherished and adored by God, and so am I. *He loves us in spite of our imperfections.* My focus needs to be placed on Him, not on my performance or perfection, because missing the mark is inevitable.

I thought that I was letting God down by not being perfect, but that's not true. That isn't what God wants me to think. It was time to celebrate life and stop attempting to live up to a miracle. Instead, He told me,

"Think on this, Helo: 'Finally, brothers, whatever is true, whatever is honorable, whatever is just, whatever is pure, whatever is lovely, whatever is commendable, if there is any excellence, if there is anything worthy of praise, think about these things.'"[2]

God hears our complaints, but He won't necessarily remove their cause. Complaining doesn't help unless it motivates us to make a change. My diagnosis, surgery, and recovery taught me a lot. I hated my diagnosis, dreaded surgery, and grumbled about the long recovery process. But then I gave thanks for great medical care, for the Great Physician, and for the miracle of life.

I was determined to take small steps forward. As Martin Luther King, Jr. once said, "If you can't fly, then run; if you can't run, then walk; if you can't walk, then crawl, but whatever you do, you have to keep moving forward." Each day, I had to choose to complain a little less and rejoice a little more.

God is patient with us. Complaining is a sign of not trusting Him. It also reveals discontent and lack of gratitude. Satan is a troublemaker and wants us to open that door of doubt and discontentment. Keep this door shut! Call on God to cover your thoughts and words. Think about this, 'Let the words of my mouth, and the meditation of my heart, be acceptable in thy sight, O Lord, my strength and my Redeemer."[3]

I am grateful that God pulled me through the surgery and recovery. He blessed me with a testimony to share. I did nothing to deserve my story. It's simply the result of His steadfast love and grace. I try not to complain about the road I have traveled; rather, I am thankful for everything God taught me.

Complaining causes damage. If we are not careful with our words and choose to speak negatively, those words become the false truth of our own and others. "Do not let any unwholesome talk come out of your mouths, but only what is helpful for building others up according to their needs, that it may benefit those who listen."[4] We shouldn't wallow in self pity, quit prematurely, or fail to seek God's best. With His help, we can learn not to complain. By God's grace, we can trust Him. I now thirst for daily time with God. It is a necessity. Quitting the complaining game helps me find hope, and with hope I can press forward with tenacity and courage.

* * *

I have learned how to lighten up, even while driving. In Seattle, some people drive like imbeciles! *People drive like crazy everywhere.* I no longer honk unless I absolutely have to. I just get out of their way, smile, pray with my eyes open, and back off politely. "*Stop kvetching about traffic, Helo. Be thankful you have a car to drive and that you are able to get behind the wheel.*"

I went shopping one day at Costco. Since surgery, it is physically difficult for me to push and fill a large cart by myself. It takes me a long time and makes me tired, but God gives me stamina and I rest in the aisles. I was determined not to complain and to do something nice for two strangers. I got to the checkout line; in front of me was a man buying turkey, bread, and milk. I quietly handed the man some cash to cover the bill. The man's response was one of thankfulness and surprise, as if he had just received a month's worth of food.

The woman behind me had three young children and one on the way. Her cart was full, the children were argumentative, and so was she. One of the children was screaming.

I stopped and asked, "Hi, could I help you for just a minute?"

Exasperated, the mom replied, "Sure, if you think you can."

I bent down, looked at her three children, and instructed, "Hey, kids, let's help Mom take the things out of the cart carefully, and put them on the conveyor belt. We can give her some rest and have some fun. Now, don't break the eggs; you will need those to help Mom make your favorite cookies."

I told the tired mom to relax and watch while each one of her three children eagerly followed my directions. They started to smile, and so did she. She then acknowledged, "You have no idea of how much you just reminded me to enjoy my day and love my children in the process."

I left the store to go home. What this woman did not realize was that she had just reminded me to patiently love my two teenage boys. I had helped her, but she had helped me even more.

On another trip to Costco, the woman behind me was purchasing over-the-counter medicine and chicken noodle soup. I quietly asked the clerk to add her soup to my bill, and then I paid and left. While unloading my items into the car, I realized that I'd forgotten to return an item, so I went back. The woman for whom I had purchased soup stopped me, thanked me for my kindness, and started to choke up.

She had moved from California to Washington because her twenty-one year old daughter had recently committed suicide, leaving behind a child of her own. This woman needed to be closer to family, so she'd left her closest friends behind. She had a family gathering to attend the next day. Normally, she made her own chicken noodle soup from scratch, but Costco's soup is just as good. She was emotionally broken and physically exhausted. She had hardly anyone to talk to. I told her that I was very sorry for her loss. We exchanged contact information and talked a few days later.

Her family gathering had gone well and so had her doctor's appointment. She wanted to know why I had bought her chicken noodle soup, and I shared my story. She told me that I uplifted her, and I humbly responded, "It's all about what God can do, not me."

I don't know what it is about shopping that leads me help others, but it has brought me to a place of complaining less about shopping. When you finish making your way through the checkout line at Costco, an employee checks your receipt on the way out. One day as I left, the woman marking receipts could not hold herself together. She looked at my cart and I handed her my receipt. I told her that I noticed her tears. "My name is Helo. I don't need to know what's going on, but I will pray for you," I assured her. She told me that one of her fellow employees was in the hospital because her brain was bleeding profusely and friends and family needed to say their goodbyes immediately.

"I know I need to," she claimed, "but I don't know how I'm going to visit her without sobbing. My heart is broken. She is an amazing woman."

I locked eyes with the woman and shared a short version of my story. I knew that it was scary to watch a friend who is about to die. I encouraged her to go see her friend, and she decided to go. I told her to focus on everything beautiful about her friend, and I promised to pray for them both. She said that she believed in prayer. I told her that hope can be found even in painful situations—through God. She stopped crying and asked if she could give me a hug. I answered, "Yes."

"Look into the eyes of the brokenhearted; watch them come alive as soon as you speak hope."

— Toby Mac

All days have beautiful moments in them as long as we refuse to focus on our troubles, and instead seek the blessings given to us. On the morning of Christmas Eve, I woke up tired because of preparations the day before. I was going to have to take a long nap. We celebrated Christmas Eve with a dinner that I'd prepared and we attended two evening church services. Immediate family and close friends understood my fatigue factor, but extended family and friends had no concept of my new normal. If I want to participate in any social activity late in the evening, I have to take a nap after lunch to replenish my energy. This cuts into my time when I'm trying to accomplish things. It's not easy, but it's easy to complain about.

Christmas morning arrived, and I was exhausted. While planning to host a large number of family members, I'd forgotten necessary ingredients for dinner, and I also needed a belated birthday gift for my nephew. The restless side of me began to surface, but I told myself, "This is the day the Lord has made, let us rejoice and be glad in it."[5]

I had no legitimate reason to complain because that day we would celebrate the birth of Jesus Christ. I drove through empty and quiet streets, thinking that not a single store would be open. Safeway was. I walked in and made my purchases.

When I feel the complaining spirit coming on, ninety-five percent of the time, I stop and pray, or do something nice for someone else. At the checkout line, I quietly asked the clerk to include the groceries of the man behind me on my bill. I paid and quickly left the store. The grocery store bagger, understandably confused while trying to pack separate groceries for me and the gentleman behind me, packed incorrectly. God had another purpose in mind.

As I started my car to leave, the man knocked on my car window. "Why did you do that for me?" he asked. I told him that this was the season to give in honor of all that God has done for us. The man told me that I had no idea how much my kind act had blessed him. He explained to me that his wife just had her fourth miscarriage that morning. They had no children yet, but desperately wanted them.

I teared up.

After a pause, I expressed my sorrow for their loss. I understood their suffering because I had gone through four miscarriages as well. He asked me how he could possibly console his wife, so we talked about how he could shower her with tender, loving care.

"Listen to her patiently, and keep telling her that you love her," I encouraged.

He asked me to stay in the car. "Please, promise not to leave until I come back. I am Muslim, and there is something very important that I must do for you." He always reciprocated kindness. I was not forcing my faith on him, and he was not forcing his faith on me. We were simply exchanging thoughtfulness.

I sat there for five minutes and used the time to pray for him and his wife. Five minutes went by quickly. My eyes were closed because I was praying in a parked car. The man knocked on my window, holding a dozen pink roses and a Nordstrom gift card that he had purchased at Safeway. He thanked me again for what I'd done, and we parted ways.

When we give to another person without seeking accolades, we eventually receive blessings. Often, we receive more than we give. I was exhausted at the idea of hosting company the next day. Although they were just things, the thought behind the roses and gift card refreshed me. They lifted my complaining heart and reminded me that I am appreciated and loved by God. How blessed I was to have children and a family to celebrate Christmas with.

*   *   *

At the start of the New Year, we were updating our kitchen. Our kitchen has recessed lighting, and we had to hang new canisters that have a halo-like trim surrounding them. I was exhausted and did not feel like driving to purchase the canisters, but the painter would be back the next day to install the lights for us, so I had to go.

It took me half an hour to get to the lighting store. I walked in and explained to the salesgirl what I needed. She went to the storeroom and came back with fourteen light canisters. I needed seventeen. I inquired if there was any way that I could pay for the other three and get them by mail. No. She told me that I could drive another fifteen minutes to get them from their warehouse, though. I explained that I tired very easily, was absolutely exhausted, and did not want to go to the warehouse.

The young clerk, in her early twenties, looked at me with tears in her eyes. She mentioned that I reminded her of her dad, who got very tired all of the time, too. He was a great person who worked hard, loved his family, and had been a triathlete, but he had been bicycling one day, been hit by a car, and sustained brain injuries. He had been through extensive physical therapy for five months but had not fully recovered. He was frustrated with not being able to run, bike, and swim like before. He complained of his legs not feeling like his own and sat in his chair for days on end, felt like he couldn't walk, and slept way too much. He was starting to become depressed. The clerk became quiet after telling me this.

I shared my story with her. I then focused on what my dad had told me about conversion-like reactions, when the brain does not communicate with the rest of the body. I told her how my dad had taught me to remedy the problem by telling my legs to move and then getting up to walk.

It turned out that her dad was a Christian, so I shared my technique of putting a Bible on the table. She was excited to hear a success story from someone else who had brain trauma, experienced similar struggles, and had found a remedy.

I never talked with this young woman again, so I don't know how things worked out for her dad, but I learned once again not to grumble. Back outside, I rested in my car for a moment to regain stamina. Then I drove to the store warehouse and picked up the extra lighting canisters. When I got home, I took a cozy nap.

My new challenge of short-term memory loss often occurs when I am fatigued or overwhelmed. I forget what has to be done, where I put an object, why I am in a room looking for something, or whether I accomplished a task in the first place. This sometimes is a nuisance, but at other times, it has silver linings.

"Did you ever stop to think, and forget to start again?"
— A. A. Milne, Winnie the Pooh

Sometimes, when I lose something, I end up organizing and cleaning parts of our home for the purpose of trying to find what I lost—then I find misplaced things that I was not even looking for. *That's a silver lining.* Sometimes, I forget what I was about to do, so I sit down, rest, and try to remember. *Rest is a silver lining.* Sometimes, when I forget what I asked my children to do, they say, "Hey, now we can be lazy for just a moment and do it later…when Mom remembers to ask us again." Then we get to smile and laugh about my memory issues. *Humor is a silver lining.*

Sometimes, I fret about my forgetfulness and think that my family must want to say, *"Please remember not to forget things!"* Often, I complain about sufferings, especially my forgetfulness, instead of looking for silver linings, or remembering everything that I am thankful for. I am thankful that God understands and adores me, despite my weaknesses.

Through it all, there is one thing that I will *never* forget. *Hope is found in God alone.* I know, without a doubt, that He is here—then I find joy amidst affliction, and reciprocate His love. God's grace helps me conquer a complaining spirit and replace it with a thankful heart. Remembering to give the glory to the One who taught me how to love Him more, and complain less, is beautiful.

Find God—and ask Him into your heart. Trust Him—and discover how beautiful it is to see Him for who He truly is. The first three stanzas of "Amazing Grace" convey the precious promise of believing:

Amazing Grace, how sweet the sound
That saved a wretch like me.
I once was lost but now am found,
Was blind, but now I see.

'Twas grace that taught my heart to fear,
And grace, my fears relieved.
How precious did that grace appear
The hour I first believed.

Through many dangers, toils and snares
I have already come;
'Tis grace that brought me safe thus far
and grace will lead me home.

—John Newton (1725–1807)

I certainly have complained about simple things, especially about my "in-house pharmacy." Sometimes, I don't feel like ingesting pills. I have a medical tray for my anti-seizure medication and my family reminds me to take my pills twice a day, every day. In addition, I have other medications for sinus issues and asthma, but I am alive and have much to be thankful for.

One night, I walked down the hallway near my bedroom, felt faint, and nearly blacked out. It felt like a 9-1-1 moment. Rich called my dad, who came over and did a full neurological exam. I just had a clear brain MRI weeks before, so there was no fear of a tumor. We discovered later that I had not taken my seizure medication for about thirty-six hours. I now fully understand the importance of taking it and will never complain about the medication again. I'm thankful that we can afford it. I'm grateful that it protects me and keeps me healthy.

I've wanted to put up a plaque in our home—"No Complaining Allowed." Instead, we have crosses hanging from just about every vantage point to remind us to be thankful for what Jesus did for us. We are all continually learning how to demonstrate gratitude. Grumbling can lead us to fall into the ditch of self pity, where Satan would like us to linger. The fact is that God has the ability to sustain us in all circumstances. He pulled me through dark discouragement with His constant presence. "You are my hiding place; you will protect me from trouble and surround me with songs of deliverance."[6]

I will do my best not to complain—with God's help.

One day, many years ago, Rich opened the door between our kitchen and garage, just like he does about every weekday around dinner time. He typically walked in and hugged me, and then the children. It was October, and we had recently celebrated my thirty-eighth birthday. He stopped, looked at me, and stated, "We need to talk."

Rich is not one to get upset easily or worry, but that night he was unusually quiet.

"Are you okay?"

"Helo, I don't have a job anymore. I've been granted six weeks of pay and some healthcare benefits, but then it is finished. This is going to be hard."

I gave him a hug and whispered, "God loves you and so do I."

"I love you too, Helo."

Rich started looking for work, to no avail. Then his job loss became less important. Rich's dad called him and revealed, "Son, I have lung cancer. The tumor is the size of a football. It's inoperable, and the doctors think I have six weeks to live." Rich spent as much time as possible with his dad over the next few weeks. We lived more than sixty miles apart. Rich would not have been able to visit his dad as often, if he'd still been employed.

His dad, Frank, endured chemotherapy, became fragile quickly, and died twenty-eight days after his diagnosis, just days before Thanksgiving. Rich, his siblings, and stepmother were all by Frank's side when he passed away. Rich loved his dad's encouragement and guidance; his dad had been his sounding board.

Christmas was quiet that year. We were sad, but found joy in celebrating the birth of Jesus Christ, our greatest gift. We placed just a few small presents under the tree. I set up a treasure hunt in our home with recycled gifts. Christmas became beautiful that night, despite our troubles, as we focused on the reason for celebration. Several months later, God blessed Rich with a job, and we learned to appreciate God's provision in new ways.

"And call upon Me in the day of trouble; I shall rescue you, and you will honor Me."

— Psalm 50:15

Rich missed his dad and began placing more emphasis on raising his own family, loving his wife, and not taking anything for granted.

God gives and takes away. Sometimes, that brings us joy. Sometimes, that hurts. In both scenarios, we can grow and see that He still loves us and never leaves our sides. Through miscarriage, Rich and I chose to be thankful for our children who are waiting for us in Heaven. We chose not to complain about unemployment; rather, we thanked God for His every provision. We chose, and will choose, not to complain about loved ones lost;

we cherish the memories we had with them. We choose not to fret about health that wavers, but give thanks for health restored. We choose not to whine about errands that need to be run or chores to be done; we are thankful that we can. We choose not to kick up a fuss about cleaning house, paying the mortgage, or doing home projects; we are thankful for the roof over our heads. We choose not to complain about the rain outside; we are thankful for umbrellas.

As parents, we choose not to quibble about our children, who sometimes challenge us; we are thankful that God gave them to us to raise. I think grown-ups do a lot of explaining and kids do a lot of complaining. Then, we switch roles, and explain and complain some more.

We choose not to be grumpy about wrinkles and hair that is turning gray, because we are thankful to grow older. As a family, we choose not to gripe about the busyness of our lives; we are thankful for the ongoing to-do list. We choose not to complain about the requests on our time by others; we are thankful for family and friends. We try to stop whimpering about everything that our delightful puppy, Buttons, chews on. She is too cute to complain about.

We choose not to complain about discouragement, and are thankful for hope found. We try not to complain when God says, "Not now" or "No." We place our trust in Him. We choose not to complain about the storms that life brings, and are thankful for the God who sustains and loves us. We choose not to focus on our mistakes and imperfections. Instead, we thank God for giving us His only Son.

Everyone in my family complains at times. But when we choose to focus on all that we have to be thankful for, finding things to complain about becomes harder—and that is good. *So we do our best to wear the "no complaining" motto on our sleeves, and it is beautifully contagious.*

Chapter Twelve

RICH IN LOVE

My beloved is mine and I am his.
— Song of Solomon 2:16 KJV —

Through physical and emotional trials, I've never forgotten how to love those close to me. My ability to love grew deeper. Now, I'm better at not taking people or things for granted.

I've always loved my family and friends, but things are much different now. When I came back home, I realized what a gift it is to be a wife, mom, daughter, sister, and friend. I'm grateful for that, and loving those around me has instilled a greater appreciation for life.

I almost did not get to stay here. I am so thankful to be able to watch my family sit together at the dinner table, do the dishes, dance in the kitchen, make messes, play basketball, run around with the dogs, decorate the Christmas tree, study hard, accomplish much, graduate from college, start law school, go for a walk, do yard work, help others, say "Mom, I love you," aspire for greatness, grow in spiritual maturity, and love Jesus.

I also love the man whom God chose for me. I am completely enamored with him. We stood before God, just over a quarter of a century ago, and exchanged our vows. At that time, we never imagined how the "in sickness and in health" portion of our commitment would draw us closer together. We have now stood through the frightening reality of "until death do us part." And whenever it makes me afraid again, Rich tells me, "Helo, neither of us knows when we're going to die, and I might go first. So, let's make the most of today, my dear." And then we do.

During the first five days of my stay in the ICU, Rich never left the hospital. For the next several weeks, he stayed with me for about ten to twelve hours each day and then went home to spend time with our two boys. He also maintained steady contact with our daughter, Lauren, who was off at college. In the ICU, he stared at the love of his life, lying there, motionless—sustained by machines. And he was afraid.

Shock consumed him.

At the start of my hospital stay, Rich did his best to maintain composure. He did not cry in front of anyone except God. He wanted to be "strong and optimistic" for our kids. Initially, he didn't turn off his cell phone because he had so many people to update continually. Then, he couldn't take or make enough calls to update people on this non-stop roller coaster situation, so he put the phone away and he focused on spending time with his Heavenly Father. God was, and is his steady sustenance.

We had chosen to share the news of my diagnosis and surgery only with family and a few close friends because we had thought the journey would be short. I'd go in for surgery, be in the hospital for six days, then come home—and we'd tell everyone about it then. Hospital admittance happened so rapidly after diagnosis, that we didn't have the time to tell very many people, anyway. We were busy getting ready. We asked our kids to keep the news in a close-knit circle because we didn't want them to have to answer countless, difficult questions, or experience the highs and lows of what we expected to be a short roller-coaster ride.

Our ways are not always God's ways—and only He knew how long the journey would be. Looking back, we realize that we should have designated friends as the "go-to" people, and kept them up to date, and they, in turn, could've updated everyone else. Instead, Rich not only stayed by my side during a difficult time, but rehearsed the details often, as he shared the updates with others.

I have asked Rich how he endured the trial of watching his wife stand at Heaven's door. He insisted that God kept him in a constant state of optimism. It was the only way that he could cope. He was absolutely exhausted and went into autopilot every day. God carried him through, and Rich's faith and trust in Jesus matured. We were both very rich in love.

I cannot imagine what it was like to watch the one closest to you lie in a coma on life support. What about all the things you had yet to do together? If we only had a few moments left to talk, what would we say?

I would say, "Rich, I love you deeply. Know that if I leave for good, I'll always be in good hands because I'll be in the arms of God. You have been an amazing, tender, and adorable husband. I'm so thankful He chose you, for me, to spend my life with. You have been and always will be an incredible father to our children. Constantly rely on God, and you'll never be alone. He loves you like no other. When you miss me, remember how much we loved each other. My comfort is found in believing that I will see you, and our children, again in Heaven."

After my journey, I fell in love with my husband much more than I previously thought possible. He and I have both been captivated by God's love. Issues that used to bother me have dissolved. I used to expect too much out of Rich, and failed at completely forgiving him for things of the past. Harboring those grudges was poisonous. When we forgive, we are emulating the character of God. Because of God's love, we can dismiss flaws in each other and love one another better. No one demonstrated true forgiveness more beautifully than Jesus; He was beaten, spit on, unjustifiably accused, and then nailed to a cross where He suffered greatly. While crucified upon the cross, Jesus said, "Father, forgive them, for they do not know what they are doing..."[1]

Rich and I are not perfect in loving and forgiving one another, but we understand the importance of forgiving and loving. We pull God into our marriage daily, and strive to love each other unconditionally. We will never be flawless at it—but it's worth striving for. I am glad to be growing old with Rich. This doesn't mean that I will never fail at showing him devotion, or that Rich is perfect at showing his love to me. Only God is perfect in love; because of Him, we are rich in love.

My husband tells me every day that I am beautiful. Rich sees many character qualities in me that he cherishes. He adores me because he sees how much I love Jesus. He keeps me humble. And he thinks, "*I am so happy that I waited for God's best. Helo is incredible.*"

I have a new normal. With the left side of my face feeling numb, it feels like that portion of my face has been removed. At times I complain, "What I wouldn't give for the left side of my face to feel like the right side of my face for even half an hour!" I often tell my husband that I'm frustrated with feeling like part of my face is not there; at times I feel deformed and ugly, and yet when I smile no one can tell.

When I feel discouraged about my face, Rich remains patient and reminds me again that I am beautiful inside and out. He points out small imperfections on his own face and body, and reminds me that I love him in spite of them. That is what true love does for one another.

Remember, God loves us in spite of our imperfections—His love is the only perfect affection.

I now tell others, "Dote on your significant others and never take them for granted." Doting does not necessarily mean giving gifts. Affection cannot be bought. It's much more than that. My husband and I have an unwritten contract on Valentine's Day; we are never to one-up each other with gifts. We only give each other a card. This started in college when we had no money. We dated for several years and married at age twenty-four. Ever since college, the rule has been—give each other only cards for Valentine's Day.

The Valentine's Day just two weeks after my surgery was difficult for my husband. He found a beautiful, red velvet card with the pearl-like embossed words "My Love" on the cover. In it, he wrote, *"Helo, you mean absolutely everything to me. Happy Valentines Day! We will celebrate when you come home. I love you very much and will always be by your side. Let us both start thinking about a fun family vacation together. And, of course, one vacation for just the two of us. You are continually in my thoughts and prayers. I will always love you, Rich."*

He read this to me out loud while I lay in a coma in the ICU. I did not respond, but Rich needed to share it, and I undoubtedly needed to hear it. I found his card a year later in a drawer with many other cards that had been given to me during my hospital stay. I read it out loud and wept. It was the first time that I'd "heard" my husband's heartfelt words.

My husband's words moved me deeply.

"You don't ever have to buy me another Valentine's Day card. In fact, you can give this one to me every February 14th," I told him.

"Are you sure?"

"Yeah, you picked out a great card and filled it with beautiful words."

He replied, "God picked out a beautiful wife for me."

"Rich, I wish that I could've reciprocated your love when you read it to me in the ICU and I'm so sorry that you had to see me that way."

"You've more than made up for it, and I never gave up on you, Helo."

Knowing that my husband never quit, despite the odds, still moves me.

A year after my surgery, we celebrated Valentine's Day again. Because I occasionally forget things, which is very common after brain trauma, I asked him every day, for about two weeks, "Where are my wedding rings?" Forgetting that I'd already asked him the day before, I asked him again. He assured me that I would find them. A girlfriend later teased, "Helo, you should have known that something was up."

Then, on February 14, 2012, Rich got down on bended knee and said, "Close your eyes, Helo." He handed me a chocolate mint. Where was the card to be given? He had just one-upped me. I only had a card to reciprocate my affection. He told me to close my eyes again, and then put my wedding rings on.

I opened my eyes and saw that my engagement ring looked different. My husband had a halo of diamonds added, to encircle the main diamond on my ring. Rich said, "God gave me my Helo back. I love you."

"Enjoy life with the woman whom you love all the days of your fleeting life which He has given to you under the sun; for this is your reward in life and in toil in which you have labored under the sun."

— Ecclesiastes 9:9

When Rich placed the rings on my finger, I cried tears of joy. The halo around my ring is beyond sentimental. It reminds me of both my husband's, and God's love for me. The diamonds mean nothing to me materialistically; their importance lies in the reminder that God placed protection around me, and miraculously, here I am today. God went ahead in the battle for me and moved the massive mountain in front of me. *Thank you, God.*

So, my friend, whoever you are, always appreciate your spouse or significant other. Dote on him or her. Be loving, patient, kind, gentle, respectful, and trustworthy. We never know when those we love will pass away. We should rejoice in each day that God gives us together.

A close college friend of mine, Kelli, lost both of her parents to a plane accident her freshman year in college. Her parents loved each other and God. Kelli's calm faith following the loss of her parents moved me in ways that I will never forget. Always love those closest to you. Cherish them and do not take your time together for granted.

Love does not lie, manipulate, tease, gossip, obsess, cling, force itself on others, purchase affection with gifts, masquerade itself, pretend, or sound sarcastic. God intentionally gives us wise instruction in the Bible on how we are to love one another.

Love is patient and kind. Love is not jealous or boastful or proud or rude. It does not demand its own way. It is not irritable, and it keeps no record of being wronged. It does not rejoice about injustice but rejoices whenever the truth wins out. Love never gives up, never loses faith, is always hopeful, and endures through every circumstance... But love will last forever.

Three things will last forever—faith, hope and love—and the greatest of these is love.

— 1 Corinthians 13:4–8, 13

My husband and I read this verse just about every week now. A plaque with this verse hangs on our bedroom wall. We sometimes insert our names in place of the word "love," reminding ourselves to love each other the way God wants us to.

I appreciate every anniversary, now, more than ever. I've gotten better at voicing my affection for my husband. I wrote this for him on our twenty-third anniversary, a little over a year after returning home:

> *You are an amazing, godly man and leader of our home. You consistently demonstrate love, gentleness, and dignity. You have a heart for growth in God. You are humble when needed and give direction with prayed-over discernment. You are an amazing father to our children. You have abundantly fulfilled our vows and have been an answer to prayer that only God could provide. You know how to celebrate joy and how to be still and strong in trials. Happy Anniversary. I love you.*
>
> — Helo

In every journey or battle, there are silver linings. For Rich, there's been the delight of the switch that was turned on during my surgery. It wears my husband out, but it's also a blessing in disguise and a problem that many married men would love to have. Prior to surgery, intimacy was often put on hold because we were preoccupied with working, running the household, and taking care of three children. Intimacy was at the bottom of the "to-do list." It was a weekly occurrence, maybe.

When I returned home, I could not get enough of my husband, in part, because I was afraid of leaving him again. I needed to be constantly close to him. I also had short-term memory loss with situations that were a common occurrence. I asked my husband for intimacy often because I could not remember when we had last been together. This left my husband exhausted.

In the past, it was usually me saying, "Not now, I am tired." Now, Rich not only says that, but goes on to say, "No, please, not this morning, not this afternoon, not this evening. Please wait. I am an older man now and need more rest between times together." Yet, he is amazed and thankful for my drive and my repeated short-term confusion in this area. A sense of gratitude and humor is helpful.

Upon visiting my neurosurgeon one day, Rich exclaimed, "I don't know how you did it, Dr. Raisis, but you are one talented doctor. You flipped a switch in my wife that I cannot turn off! She wants to be intimate all the time, and after we're together, she sometimes forgets that we just did it, and wants it again! I am too old for this."

Dr. Raisis high-fived Rich, grinned and chuckled, "Nice problem to have young man." Intimacy in a marriage is beautiful and amazing. Rich had never thought he would be a husband with the blessed problem of having to be intimate with his wife more often than he could handle.

I have learned that there are many ways to show love to my husband. In the covenant of marriage, intimacy can be a lot of fun. I've become creative and think all wives should do the same. It'd be great for a wife to surprise her husband, when he came home from work, by: telling him that the kids are all at Grandma's or a friend's house, having candles on the table, and pizza on its way; or she could surprise him by being beautifully dressed up instead of wearing everyday clothing, and tell him, "The kids are taken care of. We have dinner reservations at your favorite restaurant in half an hour. Time to go."

It is fun to show my husband sentiments of love, and he enjoys my pursuit. I never say "goodbye" to him, but rather, "See you later." Sometimes, I go to bed in my birthday suit instead of my frumpy pajamas. On occasion, when he asks me to turn on the shower for him to warm up the water (because it takes a long time in our home), I turn it on and jump in the shower and tell him that I'm warming it up for him. Gift cards to his favorite restaurant or tickets to an event he'd like to go to are other ways I like to surprise him. I've told him that Valentine's Day should be celebrated on the fourteenth of every month. It is just fun to ask him to come home for lunch with something other than food in mind. I call him, text him, or leave him a note in his briefcase, pocket, or wallet. It's always an "I love you" note and, sometimes, lists the many reasons why I adore him.

I give him a hug, a kiss, or a back rub out of the blue. I compliment his physique and character until he has heard enough. *To date, he's never heard enough.* We always have private birthday celebrations. I've surprised him with a special candlelit dinner minus the kids and then told him it would be his turn to surprise me the following week. It is a lot of fun to be surprised back by your spouse.

I shared my new habits of pursing my husband with a group of six women that I met outside of a church one day. Two, I knew well, the other four I had not yet met. We sat around a table in the sunshine, and I explained how much our husbands need to be surprised and pursued consistently.

"They will feel sought after and flattered by the love of their life, won't have any idea what just hit them, but will feel joyful. It is a gift that cannot be matched." I told these women to go home, drop everything else, surprise their husbands, and make them happy.

I've never seen six women more excited to approach a task. They told me that their husbands would be pleasantly surprised and would thank me later for the insightful instruction. I told the women that all "thank you's" should stay between husbands and wives. C. S. Lewis once wrote, "Affection is responsible for nine-tenths of whatever solid and durable happiness there is in our lives." Affection for one another is especially beautiful when we draw God into it and learn from Him how to love.

When I got home, I told Rich about my encounter with the six women at church. He offered, "It's good to practice what you preach about beautiful intimacy, my dear." And so we did. *I am so rich in love with my husband.*

Chapter Thirteen

SEVEN BLESSINGS

Remember, you are special because I made you.

— Max Lucado[1] —

Four miscarriages have left a painful footprint forever on my heart. The pain of losing children is indescribable. *"A wife who loses a husband is called a widow. A husband who loses a wife is called a widower. A child who loses his parents is called an orphan. There is no word for a parent who loses a child, that's how awful the loss is."* — Jay Neugeboren[2]

After my miscarriages, I was often reminded by other people that I could simply get pregnant again and have another child. Some people advised me to just adopt right away and get over the miscarriages. Others asked when my next infertility treatment would be. I generally did not want to talk about the issue because such conversations fueled my heartache.

When my friends talked about their current pregnancies, I wanted to isolate myself in pain; my envy of their joy just hurt. Coveting shatters the heart of the one who envies. Over time, God helped me replace the happiness I was coveting with contentment, even when I didn't have what I wanted. And one day, as time passed, my broken heart recovered, and He used what I gained from sorrow to help others.

Regarding the loss of our other children, my husband and I found, and continually find, comfort in the belief that there are four beautiful angels waiting to greet us in Heaven. God created each of them and then called them home, way too early for our liking. In contrast to this pain, stand our three, amazing, living children, whom we cherish. Lauren, my oldest, is beautiful inside and out. Jordan, my middle son, is protective, funny, and determined. Austin, my youngest child, is caring, tenacious, and bright.

God has given us deep devotion towards them. We have experienced both birth and death, celebration and tears. We love each of our seven blessings.

My daughter, Lauren, has often commented that she'd like to have a sister. There may be one waiting to greet her in Heaven. And if they are all boys, well, maybe she was meant to be our one and only favorite daughter.

All children are evidence of God's miracles. My middle child, Jordan, is certainly an example. Ten weeks into pregnancy, I began to bleed. I was terrified. An OB-GYN examined me and ran blood tests confirming that my hCG levels (pregnancy hormone) had stagnated and I was miscarrying. Levels are supposed to double every seventy-two hours. This was not the case for me.

It was a Thursday afternoon, and the doctor suggested that I go in the next day for a dilation and curettage (D&C). This is a brief surgical procedure, often done after miscarriages, in which the cervix is dilated and special instruments are used to remove tissue, lining, and embryo from the uterus.

This suggestion brought me to tears, so I asked the doctor if I could wait until Monday or Tuesday of the following week. He recommended early action to ease psychological distress and cut short the physical part of miscarriage. In addition, there was the possibility that a D&C would become mandatory, if the miscarriage did not finish naturally.

I remember the following Saturday afternoon; the sun was shining through the blinds of our bedroom windows. I got down on bended knee, sobbed, and prayed. "God, you started this creation in me—please heal the little one inside of me." I wiped away my tears and let it go. It was as if Jesus had asked me, "Helo, will you trust me?" Heartbroken and reminded of previous losses, I watched the weekend go by slowly and looked to God for comfort.

I went to the doctor's office the following Tuesday. My bleeding had tapered off and completely stopped over the weekend. I requested that my physician have my hCG levels tested again. He looked at me in disbelief but ran the test anyway. He and the other physicians could not explain why, but my hCG levels had risen to high levels; an ultrasound confirmed the viability of the pregnancy. About twenty-eight weeks later, Rich and I welcomed our son Jordan into our lives. Miracles are often difficult to explain.

*　　*　　*

No parent ever wants to watch their child or children go through immense trauma, and try as we may, we cannot always protect them from every potential anguish.

Although my husband wisely chose to guard our children until he knew what to expect, the moment arrived when my children had to visit. My husband and parents could not protect them any longer. They all wanted to see me, missed me, and wondered if I was going to be okay.

What they saw was a shock.

I was hooked up to life support, fighting for dear life. Doctors and medical staff were doing their best to keep me alive and answer the puzzling questions of: "Why? How? and When?" They never gave up. God enabled my family to persevere in hopes that I'd leave the ICU alive and my health would be restored.

My dad and mom picked up the boys and brought them to visit me. On the way to the hospital, my dad asked, "Boys, do you know what intensive care is?" Austin replied, "Everything is being done for my mom there and it's controlled with computers. There might be a lot of wires, tubes, and machines." Jordan remained silent. My dad explained what to expect, reminding them that I would be much better within several days.

The ICU was quiet and noisy at the same time: clicks, beeps, and pumping air. My daughter, Lauren, had just arrived and all three of our children walked into my room bravely and quietly with minds racing. In the stillness of the ICU, they looked at each other, then back at me, and took turns to reach out and touch my hand. I did not respond.

This was scary.

After this first visit, Lauren went back to college and our sons went home. My parents asked the boys how they felt. They somberly answered, "It was just as we had expected, only worse because it's our mom." My dad had been well qualified to prepare them for a difficult ICU situation because he had once been a hospice physician, and hospice focuses on relieving symptoms of patients and emotionally supporting their families as life fades away. But nothing could fully prepare them to see their mom on life support. *It was heart wrenching.*

My boys wanted to go back to the hospital and visit me again soon because they both hoped to see improvement. A few days later, accompanied by their sister, they walked into the ICU again.

Unfortunately, they saw no change.

A couple of weeks later, they were thankful to see minimal improvement; they got to see me smile at them and were relieved. *I don't remember this.* They tried to give me a hug, avoiding the medical wires and tubes. For my dad and husband, this was an absolute highlight.

One morning I grumbled, "Dad, I am hungry!" He jumped for joy. My appetite indicated that the brain swelling was totally gone, because a swollen brain cannot feel hungry. He shared this with my family, encouraging them.

*   *   *

My daughter was off at college, and my sons were just fifteen and twelve when I got admitted to the hospital. My sons had to grow up quickly and fend for themselves for two months while I was in the hospital with Rich by my side. They likely thought, *"We miss and love Dad and Mom. Hopefully she gets better so that they can both come back home soon. We'll just take care of ourselves for now."*

Our family went through a difficult transition when I returned home and resumed my parental role, trying to guide and discipline the boys. They lost the complete independence that had been forced upon them. It was as if they said to me, "Mom, we love you. We're glad that you are back, but when you were gone we learned how to do just about everything on our own. We don't need you to tell us what to do."

I wanted time to stand still. I wanted to hold onto every precious moment with my kids because I had come so close to not being their mom anymore. Whereas, I saw our boys as kids who had been forced to grow up too fast, they had a different perspective. They were thankful that I had survived and happy to have me home, but they were teenagers ready to spread their wings.

They seemed to be declaring, "Mom, we can call our own shots." I thought, *"Hold on a minute, boys!"* Out of a mom's love and affection, I saw that they weren't yet ready to take on the challenges of independence and freedom while simultaneously honoring their parents' instruction. It was time for Rich and me to stay strong, remain patient, and step into the gap with wisdom and love. We still do. One day, my boys will become young adults and move out on their own. Rich and I hope to look back one day, saying, "We are thankful for our three children who hold onto a strong faith in God and are raising their children to do the same." We are so blessed to be called "Mom" and "Dad" by our amazing children.

I asked my daughter to express what she went through when I was hospitalized, and here is what she wrote:

When you were in the hospital, Dad, Opa, and Oma intentionally shielded us from the seriousness of your situation. They didn't want us to fear for your safety. I understand that their intent was to protect our hearts, but I would have preferred to be more aware of the details. On my first visit to the ICU, a week after the main surgery, I walked into the hospital room and looked at you in shock. There didn't seem to be any life in you, at least not natural life. Machines were keeping you alive, and I wasn't prepared for that. I knew that you were in danger but didn't realize how much.

There was nothing to do but cry. Dad wrapped me up in a hug and whispered that everything would be okay. I didn't argue with him, but he was wrong. Obviously, we were about to lose you. Without a miraculous recovery that defied all medical logic, you were clearly about to die.

I started to run through the logistics in my mind. There would be family and friends to contact. I would first call Brenda, your dear friend since childhood, who lived across the country. She would break down in tears, and then I would cry too... Great. There would be a funeral to plan. Wait, no, Mom wouldn't want a funeral. She would prefer a "celebration of life."

There would be thank-you cards to send for all the flowers. There would be family sessions with a counselor from church. There would be the "firsts"—the first birthday, first Christmas, first graduation, first wedding, and first grandchild without Mom.

During that first visit and subsequent ones, I didn't feel much. Emotions weren't safe, so I left them outside the hospital. Numbness and busyness were my defenses, and they worked pretty well. But sometimes, I thought about the emotions that I would inevitably feel someday, if you slipped away from us. I would feel lonely. What if I got married someday and Mom wasn't there? Lonely. What if I attended graduate school, as I had always planned, and you were absent from my graduation? I'd see Dad sitting in the audience, cheering. Alone.

Another emotion was thankfulness. My brothers spent a lot of time at home. Probably lonely. Family and friends generously offered to take care of us—especially my brothers. People brought over meals, gave rides, and checked in frequently to see if there was any way to help. They were so kind, and I'm thankful that they surrounded us as a community full of hope and joy.

This sounds cliché, but God's love is what carried us through the crisis, recovery, and many months of therapy. He is our Great Counselor who comforts all who mourn and turns ashes into beauty. He doesn't give us more than we can bear in the sense that His grace strengthens us and enables us to rise up to any challenge. He is the peace for the restless, which is how I felt in the midst of suspense and powerlessness. The bottom line is that He is faithful.

And you know what? I wasn't afraid. Some might attribute my calmness to Dad's efforts to stay positive and make sure that we did the same. Others might say that my internship and schoolwork required focus; I simply had to remain calm, denying the probability of your death and shrugging off concerns. But that's not true. I wasn't afraid, because if fear crept in, I remembered and relied on God's promise that He is with us. He is always present. He holds us close to his heart, and there we don't have to be afraid.

When you were finally in the clear, I was grateful. I didn't think life would ever go back to normal, though. You might have life-long disabilities and impairments. You might have severe amnesia—at least you knew our names and faces. Well, I was wrong. You have made a full recovery in every sense of the word. I wasn't around much when you came home and started occupational, speech, and physical therapy, but whenever I did visit, you had made significant and visible progress. Mom, you are stubborn, like me.

And Mom, I may not have told you this...but I was proud of you then. I'm still proud now. You demonstrated so much resilience and courage and determination; you refused to give up. You dedicated hours every day to therapy so that you could get better for yourself and for us. Thanks for doing that. I'm proud of you. Seriously, you did a heck of a job. My hope is to be just as determined and stubborn (in the best sense) as you have been.

And Dad, you're the strongest man I know. Your faithfulness to Mom was a beautiful reflection of the faithful love that God has for us. You hardly left the hospital, served as her advocate, and held her hand for two months straight. You still haven't stopped holding her hand and being her best friend. Thanks for being the leader and friend whom we all needed.

Opa and Oma, were great too. They actually booked a hotel close to the hospital so as to be nearby and on call. Dad gets along so well with them (which isn't hard to do, because they're great). They only had one fight in two months. Opa was checking your reflexes because he's a retired doctor, and that's what he does. Dad told him to stop so that you could sleep. Oma was probably just smiling; she does that a lot.

And my brothers—well, they were brave. They had to grow up too much in two months. They got closer to each other, and they learned about compassion. Jordan would have been willing to take his mom's place, and he wasn't just saying that. He's a protective guy and a loyal friend. Austin was just waiting for you to come home, and he was really kind and helpful when you finally did. I think his sense of humor is what got him through the experience.

Since the surgery and recovery, all of us have become closer than before. I think we realized how fragile life is and instinctively grew closer to each other as a result. And since then, you have had great opportunities to encourage people in difficult circumstances. They can relate with your story, and

*they're willing to listen to how you got through: God was with
you. It's that simple.*

What Lauren wrote to me is incredible and something that I will
always cherish. When I returned home, she was away at college, where she
needed to be, but I missed her enormously. I wrote this for her:

*For my daughter, Lauren,
You are in my prayers, in my heart, and I miss you.
When I miss you, I realize how very much I love you.
When I love you, I thank my Heavenly Father for blessing me
    with an amazing daughter like you,
And then I am reminded of how much God loves each of us.
Then while I miss you, I know that He is with you abundantly.
Love, Mom*

Finally home, I got to see my boys every day. And I loved it. I remember sitting with my humble and amazing son, Jordan, one day and saying,
"Jordan, it has been a year and I haven't yet asked what you thought when
you saw me in a coma in the ICU."

He sat there, still and contemplative. Several minutes later, he replied,
"I was numb, Mom. And I wanted to take your place."

Then I asked, "If you ever had a friend who had a mom near Heaven's
gate, what would you tell them?"

Jordan said, "I would tell them that things will get better."

I learned with Jordan that sometimes it really does not take many
words to express how we feel. But it was not all sadness for Jordan. Remember that silver lining to challenges? Because of my memory loss issues, Jordan got to celebrate his sixteenth birthday twice. I forgot the first
celebration and wanted to do it again. Rich marked the second celebration
on the calendar so we would remember the event and not have to do it a
third time, even though Jordan would have been okay with that.

Jordan wrote the following for my forty-eighth birthday:

Dear Mom,

"For I know the plans I have for you," declares the Lord, "plans to prosper you and not to harm you, plans to give you hope and a future."³ That verse is my prayer for you—that no matter what, you can remember this verse and realize that God has some plans for you: Some plans of a great future, and one filled with hope!

But congratulations on continuing to be the best mother ever! Thanks for having a cheerful attitude, even with everything that you have had to deal with. I can't wait to spend many of your future birthdays with you!

Relentless determination
Strong belief in Christ
Funny
Always ready to evangelize
Cheerful spirit
Servant's heart
Encouraging
Loving
Strong teacher
Selfless
Resilient
Gracious

Those things are just the tip of the iceberg of why you are amazing.
So Happy Birthday, Mom!!!
Love you,
Jordan

Austin was only twelve when this all happened and was likely the most confused and afraid. He thought that I would return home in six days. Eight weeks passed, and that worried him.

"One day he and I would laugh together again, right?"

God gifted Austin with a great sense of humor and the ability to find reprieve in difficult situations. He was the one who was born after six weeks of mandatory bed rest on my part. He once told me that my bed rest was him giving me the gift of a six-week vacation.

When I was pregnant with Austin, the placenta was in a precarious place right over the cervix, and I could've easily miscarried. I was required to rest horizontally until he grew and the uterus expanded. The placenta would then move to a safer place away from the cervix, reducing the risk. At first, bed rest was tough because I was restless and jittery, wanting to jump right out of bed. After several days, my muscles began to atrophy and the feeling of restlessness went away.

I didn't have to cook, clean, or be a busy mom during that time. We hired my sister-in-law's sister, Janice, as a nanny to take care of the kids. While on bed rest, I got to hear the kids having fun and playing in the inflatable pool outside. Splashing is a fun noise to listen to. I got to smell delicious pancakes every morning, which was delightful. Listening to my children play, took away my frustration of having to stay in bed for six weeks. Austin, you were worth every moment of bed rest. Thank you for the six week vacation. I love you!

Austin weathered the storm of my brain surgery in his own way. When I finally came home he greeted me with a hug and a stack of Post-it® Notes. On them he had written:

"Read all of these to make 'you' feel better."

"Have I not commanded you? Be strong and courageous. Do not be frightened or dismayed, for the Lord your God is with you— always."[4]

"If I could have chosen the word for perfect, it would have been you."

"For You will light my lamp. The Lord will lighten your darkness."[5]

"His hand will lift you up."

"I LOVE YOU, MOM!!!!"

"You have been fearfully and wonderfully made by God."

"You are the best thing that has happened to me."

"I Love You—It is true—You I Love—Love you I do"

On my next birthday, Austin wrote me this note:

I don't know what I would do without you in my life. You're so caring and considerate and really try to do what's best for me. I love you so much and I hope you have an awesome birthday and upcoming birthdays!!!!!!!!!!!! I'm really fortunate to have someone like you for a mom. Happy Birthday! Love, Austin

I don't let a single day go by without telling my children that I love them. My seven blessings are amazing—those here on earth, and those waiting to greet me in Heaven.

Chapter Fourteen

AVALANCHE OF Post-it® Notes

Let the words of my mouth and the meditation of my heart be acceptable in Your sight, O LORD, my rock and my Redeemer.
— Psalm 19:14 NASB —

My husband and I have always enjoyed leaving notes for each other. When he travels, I leave messages in his wallet or suitcase. He reciprocates by leaving notes in our bedroom, bathroom, or closet to let me know that he will miss me while out of town. Rich sometimes leaves messages for me and the kids in plain view. Other times, he hides them to surprise us.

When our kids were young and went off to church or sports camp, we placed notes in their suitcases. We flooded them with messages of love and verses of encouragement. The avalanche of Post-it® Notes subsided as they got older because it became embarrassing for them to open up their suitcase in front of their cabin mates and hear, "Oh, your mommy loves you!" But we would include at least one note to remind them how much they were loved. The notes keep coming as they get older: "I am proud of you," "I love you," "God loves you," "Have a great day!" "Hope the exam goes well," and "Congratulations on a job well done."

Because of my short-term memory loss following surgery, I needed reminder notes just about everywhere—notes reminded me of the things that I should not forget, but then I'd forget where the Post-it® Notes were placed. At first, this was confusing, but later, it was beneficial. Leaving Post-it® Notes retrained my brain to remember things.

Before diagnosis and surgery, my husband and I sketched our future, and planned things that we wanted to do as a couple and as a family. As a busy wife and mom, I wrote an ongoing to-do list daily. I once complained to my mother-in-law that I always had a never-ending list of to-dos. She reminded me to be thankful that I was alive to fulfill my list of orders. If the list permanently disappeared, that meant I wasn't around anymore. Sometimes I added tasks to my to-do list right after accomplishing them so I could cross something off; I needed to feel a sense of accomplishment. As a mom, I sometimes felt taken for granted, so checking things off the list was a personal reminder that I was doing a good job.

After returning home from the hospital, my husband and I left more Post-it® Notes than before. Our appreciation for each other grew exponentially. We no longer communicated during our busy days the way we used to via texts, voice mails, and e-mails; it needed to go deeper than that. Rich left Post-it® Notes for me on top of my pillow, on the bathroom mirror, in my car, in my makeup drawer, in my purse, or in my coat pocket, and I would reciprocate.

I once told close girlfriends about this. One responded, "Well, at least you have a husband who adores you! You also have a legitimate excuse for memory loss, and a reason for putting Post-it® Notes every-where. I forget things all of the time, and can't remember why or where I put the notes to remind me what to do."

Post-it® Notes have many purposes. Forgetfulness is not easy to deal with. It confuses the best intentions and complicates goals. It can be embarrassing, too. But by God's grace, it is tolerable, and sometimes funny. The key is to never forget about Jesus. He makes it possible to withstand adversities without giving up hope.

I left notes in the car to remind me when and where I had to pick up or drop off my kids. I put notes in the bathroom and kitchen, reminding me to take medications. Over time, I discovered that leaving notes everywhere improved my ability to remember.

I even had to write reminder notes about the dogs. I used Post-it® Notes on the laundry room door to remind me where the pet supplies were. This jogged my memory to give the dogs their medications, to groom them, or to buy a new leash when Buttons had chewed another one to shreds. (Everything in the house is a tasty chewtoy for Buttons: Jordan's deodorant, Rich's favorite slippers, ceramic salt and pepper shakers, magazines, batteries, electrical chords, needles and thread, unopened paper towel rolls, my new dress, and needlepoint pillows with feathers inside of them.) Buttons has expensive taste.

Leaving Post-it® Notes for one another can be fun! One day, my husband worked from home. His office is located in our bedroom and he asked not to be bothered because he had a lot of work to do. I ignored his request and handed him a note: "Time to get it on and practice what Helo preached about beautiful intimacy." Rich smiled and said, "I love you, but I am very busy with work. Leave me alone now, and put the note by the bed." He watched me put it by his side of the bed and told me to move it to my side; he did not need the reminder, but I might. I smiled, remembering that I was the forgetful one between the two of us, put the note on my side of the bed, and gave him a hug. He continued working without further interruption.

We now have a rule that he will inform me of the hours of his conference calls when he's at home. I don't disturb him because a Post-it® Note is placed on the outside of our bedroom door which read, "Do Not Disturb." I seldom get to interrupt Rich when he works from home, but I don't complain. He works hard to provide for our family. His company gave him two months off while I was hospitalized, and for that, we are thankful.

The "Do Not Disturb" Post-it® Note on our bedroom door has dual benefits for both work and time alone together. Late in the evening if our door is closed, our kids read it and leave us alone, or knock on the door if they really need us.

When I returned home after eight weeks of hospitalization, encouraging notes were placed everywhere. I was thankful to be home but spent the majority of the day asleep in bed. On the wall above my pillow, a Post-it® Note read, "God hears our every prayer even when we whisper." On my nightstand, I put a note: "Rise and shine and give God the glory, Helo. You are alive and He is alive in you." On my bathroom mirror, a Post-it® Note said, "Helo, be still and know that God is who He said He is. He stayed by your side through the worst of this ordeal and He will love and strengthen you through the rest of it." On my bedroom mirror, "God remind me to remember how much you love me." On my bedroom door, another note declared, "Helo, you can do all things through Jesus who gives you the courage, tenacity and strength to endure affliction." Some messages were short: "Never quit."

There were times when I ripped the notes to pieces in frustration. New Post-it® Notes of encouragement were written: "Find hope," "Trust God," and "It is His battle." On the refrigerator, a note displayed: "It is okay that there is no ice cream, because a healthy diet is important." This one was taken down frequently by our children. I wanted to place a Post-it® Note, "Eat your vegetables."

When I first got home, walking a few steps was hard. I walked into walls, felt like a teeter-totter, couldn't balance well, and all the walls looked crooked because of my contorted, constant, double vision. I put a Post-it® Note on the banister saying, "He makes crooked ways straight."[1] Over time, He did.

After a while, my doctor gave me the go-ahead to walk on a treadmill. On it, I placed a Post-it® Note that said, "Helo, you can do it because God has this challenge in His grip!" Walking on the treadmill was scary because I still wobbled when I walked, and lack of constant balance challenged me. In frustration, I ripped down the note of encouragement; the next day, I replaced it, motivated to press on. Now I walk the treadmill almost daily.

I have found hope and a new daily walk with God. Post-it® Notes conveyed messages of encouragement and inspiration, and the reminders retrained my brain and lifted my spirit. On one I wrote, "Cherished one,

You can do all things through Christ who loves you and gives you the strength to go on."[2]

One day, my children started using Post-it® Notes, too. They stuck messages on walls and ceilings for each other. It brightened my day and made me giggle and smile. In Austin's room, Lauren placed one on his dresser. It read, "How to put on pajamas: 1. Put them on 2. Fold and put away clothes." The one on the light switch by his door read: "Say your prayers." On a picture of a renowned basketball player doing a slamdunk: "Be a better person tomorrow than you were today." On the headpost of his bed: "Sleep well."

Then Austin posted remarks in Lauren's room. By a lamp at the side of her bed; the Post-it® Note read, "Nighty-night." On the mirror hanging by her closet he wrote: "Girl, you is purty!" One of my favorites is the one he put on the wall in her room: "Be nice to thy brother, New Testament something." And his sense of humor just had to put one on the ceiling: "I don't know how I did this; God must have helped me."

In the bathroom, Lauren put up more Post-it® Notes. Above the sink, she commented: "How to wash your hands: 1. Flush the toilet, 2. Wash hands, 3. Congrats!" In fine red print, she had written, "Caution: Don't touch sign—trouble will come upon you!" Above the toilet, she posted: "Stop! Did you flush the toilet?" Days later, above the toilet, Lauren put up a card depicting a face with googly eyes and a Post-it® Note that commanded, "Flush Me!" And in fine red print: "Do not remove." Days later, Jordan replaced that note with his own: "Challenge Accepted!" Lauren replaced his note then with "Flush the Freakin' Toilet, you Hooligans!" The response, days later: "Oh bummer, call a plumber!"

Austin put notes on the shower, including "No singing permitted. Ever! Unless you are awesome. Seriously though, like me. Legendary..." Later, he placed another Post-it® Note on the shower: "Don't forget to take off your socks before entering." I wanted to post under this: "Unless you are planning to multitask and wash your socks in the shower so that Mom will have less laundry to do."

And so we keep leaving Post-it® Notes. It makes us smile and brings us joy. We are blessed with communicating with one another. Face-to-face conversations are the best, but life gets busy, and so, moving forward, we will always enjoy this avalanche of Post-it® Notes.

Chapter Fifteen

A PARENT'S SUFFERING

He will wipe every tear from their eyes,
and there will be no more death
or sorrow or crying or pain.

— Revelation 21:4 NLT —

Combine the devotion of every parent who cherished, cherishes, or will cherish his or her child on this planet. Stop and think about how staggering that collective love would be. God's love is infinitely greater than all of that devotion combined. Now that is one—amazing—love. The potential of losing a child is painful, and the loss of a child is heartbreaking. There is no specific schedule for time needed to heal and I don't believe that the pain of loss ever completely vanishes—but with God, suffering is tenderly understood.

"Children are not supposed to die...Parents expect to see their children grow and mature. Ultimately, parents expect to die and leave their children behind...This is the natural course of life events, the life cycle continuing as it should. The loss of a child is the loss of innocence, the death of the most vulnerable and dependent. The death of a child signifies the loss of the future, of hopes and dreams, of new strength, and of perfection."[1]

As parents, we sometimes watch our children suffer in big or small ways. When toddlers stumble and fall, we encourage them to get up and walk again, courageously. When we watch them lose their way, it often hurts us more than them. One day, I took my five-year-old daughter shopping. I was holding her hand, but let go for a moment to pull something off of the rack. In a moment, she was gone, lost, or taken. If she thought we were playing hide-and-seek, it was not funny. I called security immediately. They announced her name over the loudspeaker, telling her to go to a cash register and tell someone that she was there. We still could not find her. I started calling her name, hoping to get a response. Finally, I heard, "Mommy, I am right here."

Relieved, I asked her, "Where, Lauren?"

She said, "I'm hiding in a circle of clothes on hangers."

"Come out, Lauren."

"No, Mommy. It's fun in here."

There were too many roundabout hangers in the store for me to find her, so I replied, "Okay, Lauren, keep talking to me so that I can find out where you are having fun."

She kept saying, "Here I am, Mommy." I found her in the spot where we originally started shopping.

"Lauren," I inquired, "Why did you hide in here and not come out when I called you?"

She said, "Well, hiding in here is a lot of fun. I heard you call me a couple of times, but then I heard someone that I did not know call my name. I kept hiding because you and Daddy told me not to talk to strangers. So I didn't. Then I heard you, Mommy. Here I am."

We hugged. I was elated that she'd been found so quickly and easily. *Imagine God's joy when He sees that we understand what it means to be no longer lost, but found.*

When Jordan was just learning how to ride a tricycle, I did not want him to fall and get hurt, so I made him wear a helmet. He was having fun, and I enjoyed watching him. I sat down with my lemonade. It was a warm, sunny evening. Suddenly, I heard squawking and shrieking. A big black bat, attracted by the squeaky tricycle, was dive-bombing my son.

The bat got so close that Jordan accidentally ran over it, and it got stuck under his wheel—but was still alive. I was thinking that the bat would bite my son. The mother bear in me came out.

I exclaimed, "Jordan, get off the bike and run into the house."

He laughed and protested, "But Mom, the bat is cool."

"No it isn't, Jordan. Just because you think something is cool, doesn't mean it is a good idea to play with it. That bat probably has rabies and could bite you and make us both crazy," I told him. I pulled him off his tricycle, and we went into the house to be safe.

An hour later, Jordan wanted to go back out on his tricycle, and the noise attracted the bat again. This time when it attacked Jordan, I called my husband outside. He told us to go back in. We watched him from the window. His innovative solution was to run around like crazy, yell, and swing a baseball bat at the bat. That didn't work, so we oiled the tricycle's wheels, and the squeakiness disappeared. The pesky bat never returned.

As Jordan and my other children grow older, and as long as I get to be their mom and my husband gets to be their dad, we will continue to remove the squeakiness from bad situations by oiling them with wisdom and protection. It is an honor to be our children's parents. We will tell them to draw near to God as they face different challenges and decisions in life.

Likewise, God must want us to have faith and notice that He is walking with each of us, and He promises not to leave us. Hope, wisdom, peace, and faith can be found in all circumstances when Jesus is called to our side.

Once, in the middle of the night, I learned what it means to be a frightened mom who needs to ask God for peace. My daughter had a tonsillectomy at the age of eighteen. Complications are rare with this type of surgery, but a week into the recovery, she woke up in the middle of the night, bleeding. A scab had come off the back of her throat, tearing an artery. My husband grabbed towels. We jumped into the car and rushed to the emergency room, where we learned that our daughter had lost a dangerous percentage of her blood volume. The ER doctor told us, "An emergency operation needs to be performed immediately to stop the bleeding, pump her stomach, and save her life. The doctor who has been called in to perform the surgery will talk with you both shortly."

An Ear, Nose and Throat (ENT) physician, with a nurse standing by his side, stopped in the hallway, right outside the surgical suite doors, to talk with me and Rich while Lauren lay on an ER transfer bed right next to us. It was time for her to be wheeled into surgery for the urgent procedure. The ENT asked if we would prefer to have Lauren airlifted to the local children's hospital. This doctor hadn't done the original tonsillectomy, and apparently, he did not want to assume liability.

I've been around a lot of doctors in my lifetime and am not afraid to speak my mind when addressing them—and good doctors listen, "Right Dad?"

"Doctor," I challenged, "Would you not agree that time is of the essence?" He agreed, but responded in a reserved, conversational manner. I remember grabbing the surgeon by the arm before he entered the operating room and telling him, "Get straight in there and save my daughter's life."

The nurse saw my concern and promised to update us often. It was about three o'clock in the morning when Lauren went in for surgery; my husband and I were frightened and exhausted. We went to a quiet waiting room and prayed. We received updates every fifteen minutes for more than an hour and a half; it felt like forever to me. I paced and prayed, paced and prayed, over and over again. It is difficult for any parent to see their child suffer; it is tough to wait to hear if your child is going to be okay.

Waiting can be excruciating.

Finally, our hearts stopped racing when the doctor opened the door to the waiting room. Dressed in surgical clothing, gloves off, with a look of relief on his face, he told us, "Lauren survived. She is going to be okay and is being moved to the recovery unit right now." Rich and I hugged each other and thanked God. We got to hold and hug our daughter in recovery about thirty minutes later. Words cannot describe how beautiful and precious that moment was.

After having that experience, I can only imagine how hard it was for my parents to watch me suffer with my brain tumor removal. I asked my mom what it was like to have her daughter go through this. For her, the ordeal started when she received my call about the initial diagnosis, and she and my dad had to come pick me up at the doctor's office. When she saw me there, sitting on that curb, in the rain she went into a complete state of shock and hardly knew how she got to my home.

Later, when I was wheeled into surgery, she said that life felt surreal for her. Having great confidence in the doctor's ability, and believing I would be back home soon did not prepare her for what she saw that first time in the ICU. Her daughter was a determined fighter, but was not "okay."

While I was on life support, Mom attempted to count the wires and tubes connected to my body. She lost track at forty. Later the number of wires and tubes almost doubled, as far as she could tell.

One of the worst moments for my mom was when she came to visit me and learned that I had almost died earlier that morning. She asked the nurse why she, my dad, and husband had not been informed as soon as *Code Blue* had been called. The nurse explained that it all had happened too fast; medical staff had rushed in to surround me. First, they had to keep me alive. After doing so, they saw no reason to call my parents and husband at two a.m., wake them up, and explain the situation. They thought everyone needed rest. For my mom and my dad, this entire situation was a nightmare. After that, they were hesitant to leave the hospital for fear that another *Code Blue* would be called in their absence, preventing them from saying their final goodbyes.

Now it was even harder for my mom to visit me, because she was expecting the worst. Yet, she continued to visit me daily, talking to me in my comatose state, regardless of whether I could hear it, because she felt a connection between us. She needed it, and I did, too. She talked to me every day, believing that God was talking to me on one side—and that I could hear her talking to me on the other. She would come in and say, "Hi, Helo! I love you," and then ask how I was doing. She did this daily, in spite of the fact that I didn't respond for weeks.

I was placed between blankets of ice to induce hypothermia, in an effort to rid my brain of swelling. My mom would grab my icy toe, wiggle it, and say, "Hi, Helo." She talked to me every day during my ICU stay, not expecting me to answer. Then one day, I surprised her. She looked at me, saw that my eyes were shut and my body was still and said, "Hello, Helo, I will always love you." I slowly lifted my right hand just a few inches and slowly turned my wrist. Then my hand quickly dropped back down. That was my wave. *My mom was ecstatic.* I had finally communicated after being comatose for weeks. She immediately told the rest of family what she had just seen, and they were overjoyed.

Through everything, my dad never thought he would lose me. Like my husband, my dad was optimistic—perhaps overly so. It was a coping mechanism. He insisted that I would come home again but worried about my condition. *"Will Helo end up vegetative?"* The tumor was on the left side, and he knew the left side of the brain manages communication. He wondered, *"Will she talk again?"* The brain also controls the ability walk; *"Will she end up paralyzed?"* And being near the optic nerve, he had to wonder, *"Will she lose her sight?"* Those thoughts were agonizing for my dad.

As the team wheeled me into the operating room, my father watched closely. Then his heart had become heavy and tears had welled up in his eyes. All he could think was, *"Please, God, let this go all right."* He hoped for me to be fully functional and not severely disabled.

During the surgery, my dad's mind wandered into the operating room: seeing the anesthesia being induced, my head being prepped and mechanically strapped down, and my body secured into place. He was marking time. He saw Dr. Raisis' scrubbed hands, now with gloves on, instruments ready and lights adjusted. He waited, letting his mind drift, letting more time pass. My dad felt numb and held his wife tightly. When my mom asked, "How do you think it is going?" He tried to reassure her as best as he could. But he couldn't help imagining Dr. Raisis making an incision in my scalp and preparing to cut the skull next. That was too much for my dad; he had to let go of the imagery. He quieted his mind and let time pass.

After what seemed like a long while, the silence was interrupted by the first phone call from the medical staff: "Everything is going well. We will continue to keep you posted every hour." My mom got herself a cup of coffee. My dad tried to sleep some time away. This did not work. Time went by slowly, so my dad stopped looking at his watch over and over again. He imagined incisions being made, tissues being identified and retracted, X-rays being taken for localization, suctioning to keep the operative site dry, cauterizations, and the exposure of the brain. He knew the tumor was deep inside the brain and they had to be very careful not to injure the surrounding tissue.

Then my dad did not want to think anymore. He could have handled the imagery as a physician, but not as a dad. He talked to himself as if to me: *"Helo, I love you, and you will be okay. You are in the best of hands."*

Another phone call came: "Everything is going very well with no complications at all." He felt reassured but still cautious.

There were three deep sighs of relief. Four hours into surgery, my dad ventured to let his mind peek back in. They must be extracting the tumor. He became nervous and started shaking. It was a large tumor on the cavernous sinus, a very sensitive structure with lots of small blood vessels, and he thought, *"I hope my daughter does not lose too much blood. Please, God, help me. I must trust You now."* His suffering began to consume him. He could not eat or rest, being absorbed with worry.

Another phone call announced, "All is going very well; we are getting ready to close the skull. The doctor will come by within an hour." It was now six hours into the main surgery. Finally, a knock on the waiting room door. The anesthesiologist came in to say that everything had gone well. My dad asked if the tumor was out. "Yes. All of it!" announced the anesthesiologist. "Dr. Raisis will be out shortly."

My family could finally breathe again.

The door opened, and an exuberant Dr. Raisis walked in with a large folder in his hand. "We were very lucky. We got it all. Helo will be fine." He opened the folder and started to hand out photos of the various stages of the surgery. There were pictures of the operative site, the cavernous structure with multiple cauterizations, and finally, the tumor all alone, enclosed in a jar. Dr. Raisis believed that I had a strong chance of surviving and being physically restored.

An hour later, my parents and husband visited me in the ICU. They had me back. At least for a while. I have been blessed by how much my parents love me and how they continually stayed by my side. They ached while watching me suffer—the kind of suffering that makes a parent wail inside.

I often stop and think about how much our Heavenly Father loves us. Watching us ache and suffer, in adversities and sin, must make Him sad. He sacrificed His one and only beloved Son out of His perfect love for us. He watched His Son suffer as He was mocked, spit upon, beaten, and nailed to a cross to be crucified for the sole purpose of our redemption and salvation, "For God so loved the world, that He gave His only begotten Son, that whoever believes in Him shall not perish, but have eternal life."[2]

Chapter Sixteen

PUZZLES

And we know that God causes all things to work together
for good to those who love God, to those who are
called according to His purpose.
— Romans 8:28 NASB —

Playing a part in one of God's miracles of healing is humbling and overwhelming because I did not deserve, or earn it. If God chooses to heal, it has nothing to do with me, anyway. As I see others suffer, I hope that they will pull through and see brighter days ahead no matter what today has in store for them—or what tomorrow brings. Worrying does not remove tomorrow's afflictions or troubles, instead, it takes away today's thankfulness and joy. I pray that those in the midst of trouble will not be shaken to a place of wanting to quit, and that they will see that God knows how to hold unto each of us and equip us to be brave. I suffered a lot, but I survived. I wonder, why do some suffer and die way before their time?

Heaven waits for us, and peace is found there, but suffering here still hurts. I wonder, *"Why me, God?"* because I am puzzled as to why He chose to heal me and not someone else. I have always thought of myself as a humble person, but not like I do now. "Humble yourselves, therefore under the mighty hand of God so that at the proper time He may exalt you."[1] I have repeatedly asked God to show me what He wants me to do with *His* story. This is not mine. I will not boast. All accolades go to Him alone.

A few years before my brain tumor removal, I embraced a dear friend, Brenda, and her family. Brenda and I met in high school and have been friends ever since. She became a nurse and married Russ, whom she met in college. Russ was much like my husband: driven, compassionate, humble, patient, and handsome. But most of all, he was a man who loved God genuinely. His faith created character qualities that caused him to be loved by many.

Russ had just completed his studies in cancer biology and preventative nutrition when he moved his family to Ohio, where he had accepted a position as a cancer-prevention research scientist. Everything that Russ had worked so hard for was beginning to pay off. Brenda and Russ had three beautiful children and a fourth, Christopher, on the way. For months, the family prepared for their son's arrival. Bringing Christopher into the world was going to be beautiful. And it was.

Just one month after Christopher was born; Russ became very tired and attributed it to having a newborn. But the real reason for Russ' fatigue was acute erythroid leukemia, an aggressive form of cancer. I'll never forget when Brenda called me. She was panicking. Russ was only forty-three years old. My dear friends and their entire family were in a terrifying situation. I prayed continually and asked God to be their strength.

"Mercy unto you, and peace, and love, be multiplied."
— Jude 1:2, KJV

Russ' prognosis was frightening. As a cancer research biologist, he understood the risks of medical treatment options, but was willing to do anything to get rid of the leukemia. He spent more time in the hospital enduring aggressive treatment than at home. He placed himself in the fortress of God and was an unbelievable inspiration to me, and many others. Although physically weak and suffering, Russ found strength because he put his trust in God. "And after you have suffered a little while, the God of all grace, who has called you to his eternal glory in Christ, will himself restore, confirm, strengthen, and establish you."[2] God knows how to make us strong.

Russ often rested in the lyrics of the song, "Strong Tower" by Kutless. Here is a portion of them:

In the middle of my darkness
In the midst of all my fear
You're refuge and my hope
When the storm of life is raging
And the thunder's all I hear
You speak softly to my soul

Chorus

> *I go running to your mountain*
> *Where your mercy sets me free*
>
> *You are my strong tower, shelter over me*
> *Beautiful and mighty, everlasting King*
> *You are my strong tower, fortress when I'm weak*
> *Your name is true and holy and Your face is all I seek*

Russ fought hard for ten months. I flew out to Ohio twice, with my daughter Lauren, to see him and his family. The first visit was in the summertime, right after his bone marrow transplant. Weeks after searching for a match, a bone marrow donation was flown across the ocean to help Russ fight. Feeling better for even a short time was an amazing gift to encourage Russ and his family to press forward. They cherished that time of "remission" together. When remission ended, pain and fear returned. I did not want to hear that his family was going to lose him. I cried out, *"Dear God, no!"*

The second time my daughter and I flew to Ohio, it was for Thanksgiving. We sat around the table and enjoyed one another's company. Russ made the effort to join us around the table. I could see that he was tired and didn't feel hungry, but he wanted to be with his family. A couple of days later, I remember walking into his room where he laid comfortably. He simply said, "Helo, you got here just in time." He knew something that the rest of us did not yet know.

Lauren and I spent the days helping with the children, running errands, and cleaning the home. Our favorite moments were reading and playing with the kids. Russ' mom was there too, and his brother was on the way.

Shortly after Thanksgiving, I watched Russ make his way down the stairs with Brenda's help to go to the hospital. Chemotherapy was waiting for him. He returned home weaker than before he left. *He was exhausted and fragile.*

Brenda is one of my dearest friends. She dealt with Russ' affliction by living in an eternal state of optimism, waiting and believing that God would provide a last-minute miracle. I did not fully understand her at the time, especially when looking at Russ' condition. He was weak and emaciated. Now I understand why Brenda handled the potential of losing her beloved Russ in the way she did. The revelation came to me when I learned how my husband depended upon optimism and his faith to cope with my medical crisis.

In the early morning hours on the first day of December, Brenda listened to Russ' heartbeat. It beat quickly, and she was certain that this was the last-minute miracle for which she had prayed. She called for their three oldest children, getting them in the middle of the night. I will never forget seeing the unbelievable joy in the children as they thought that this was God's miracle taking place.

But then Russ stopped breathing. He lay there in uninterruptible stillness and passed into Heaven. God was Russ' fortress when he was weak. Within moments, I was the one feeling the panic; I was at a complete loss as to how to console Brenda and her children. I had just watched an amazing husband and father die. There I stood, by his precious wife and their beautiful children, in the middle of the anguish of their loss. It hurt so much to watch, so I called out to the One who I knew could help them. In my prayer, I found rest and understood that only God could meet them in their sorrow. When someone leaves us, it feels unreal, and we find ourselves waiting for them to come home. *But they don't.* God understands firsthand how painful it is to watch a loved one die; He watched his only Son suffer and die on the cross.

Brenda later looked back at her "optimism" as denial at the thought of losing Russ, but she never gave up on God's undeniable ability to heal. And He did, in His way, for His purpose. Russ is in a safe place now, completely void of pain. He is with Jesus, down upon his knees, worshipping God, then up and dancing in celebration. My daughter and I helped Brenda, her children, and her extended family through their agonizing journey of losing a husband, dad, son, brother, uncle, and brother-in-law in Russ. Russ has been, and will continually be missed by many, but our peace comes in knowing exactly where he is.

God used Russ' story to prepare me for a terrifying journey that I never saw coming. When pain and tragedy hits, His monumental love never fades away or gives up. Years later, I told Brenda how Russ had inspired me to press on, and she replied, "Oh, my dear friend, now we can step back and look at the big picture—what a tapestry God is weaving! I am so thankful He is using my thread to weave yours and your thread to weave mine. Thank you for sharing this. I love you."

"Although this world is full of suffering it is full also of the overcoming of it."

— Helen Keller

The humbleness factor sets in when I ask myself, "Why Russ and not me?" This is a question that only God can answer. Russ instilled in me a tenacity to seek after God for courage and strength. God gives, and He takes away. He has a reason for it all. Life is a spectrum. Some have it hard and some have it easier. I have a few friends or family members who seemingly skate through life, or at least hide adversity well. But the overall majority has, or will face affliction: Cancer, loss of a child, unemployment, financial struggle, divorce, infidelity, depression, death of someone close or unexpected catastrophe. The common thread is that all of us experience difficulty. The only thing worse than the difficulties we face is the attempt to go through them by ourselves—without God.

"I lift my eyes to the mountains—Where does my help come from? My help comes from the Lord, the Maker of Heaven and earth."

— Psalm 121:1-2

I have *no idea* how people do it without God. It's poignant to see people who do not know Him, cry out in anguish to Him when devastation hits. He is always there at that moment. But He's also there in between life's challenges. When we get to know and love Him, He makes life beautiful through the good times and equips us with strength through the bad. With God all of us can endure. With God we are redeemed. With God our suffering will one day pass—when we enter Heaven. Until then, cherish each day here. That's what losing Russ taught me.

"I have fought the good fight, I have finished the race, I have kept the faith."

— 2 Timothy 4:7

I met my dear friends, Tim and Diane, during Russ' struggle with cancer. Tim is a Professor Emeritus of Cellular and Molecular Medicine, College of Medicine, at the University of Arizona and was Russ' mentor. Diane and I call each other Salt and Pepper because she has light hair, and I have dark. We are complementary. We have been friends for several years, but it feels like we've been dear friends for a lifetime. Tim is a superlative scientist, mentor, and an honored man in the cancer research community. He is a man of few words, but when he does speak, he inspires many. My husband and I have the privilege of knowing both Tim and his beautiful wife Diane, well. And we love them.

Several years ago, Tim was diagnosed with Parkinson's disease (PD). I am puzzled as to why God would allow such an incredible couple to personally face the challenge of PD when they are such contributors in the race to find a cure for cancer. They are beyond compassionate, always humble and generous.

Why do bad things happen to good people? Why do good things happen to bad people? Good and bad things do not discriminate. They happen. The reality is that everyone is tainted with sin. All of us are "bad" at times. None of us are perfect at being "good," and even if we attempt to hold ourselves to a high moral standard, it does not mean that bad things will not happen to us. Life is puzzling—we live in a fallen world and one day God will answer all of our questions. *Then we will understand.*

*   *   *

Tim and I talk often about what it's like to have a disability or illness that affects the brain. People will tell us both that we look great, but on the inside we have physical, cognitive, and emotional challenges. Sometimes we feel trapped inside our bodies, and no one other than God really understands. But when Tim and I talk to each other about our complex struggles, there is an instantaneous understanding because our challenges parallel each other. This is encouraging. We can console each other without facing the arduous task of having to explain how we feel or have felt. Our combined mottos are: *pray, focus, persist, have faith, and never give up.*

Tim effectively deals with the challenges of Parkinson's disease through his faith in God, sense of humor, medication, and an exercise program through PWR!Gym® and the PD-specific foundational exercises, PWR!Moves™.[3] Focus is placed on big and fast movements and improving overall function. The goal is to help those with PD get better and stay better. Motor control, rigidity, and freezing are among the multiple symptoms of

PD addressed. It is problematic for people with Parkinson's to connect sequences to complex behaviors.

Tim is also well acquainted with fatigue and it doesn't easily leave him. Exhaustion interrupts his passions but does not erase them. For me, I tire easily, but my mornings start out well after a full night of rest. I suppose this is because my brain had time to rest and recuperate from the tasks of the day before. In my "new normal," my brain can only handle so much stimulation housed in one of three areas: emotional, physical, and cognitive. *Brain trauma opens the door to the daily introduction of exhaustion.* If I overdo it in any one of these three areas, I crash by dinner time or early evening. Then my "off times" begin, because my stamina is not the same as it was before surgery. I've learned that evenings are significantly extended if I nap during the day. So, I nap often.

Tim has told me, that during his "off times" when dealing with Parkinson's he can hardly move his limbs. He needs help getting dressed and walking. These "off times" can happen with no warning, which makes for some amusing situations. One day, he went to a restaurant in Tucson and froze in a bathroom stall. His wife had to send in some male friends to find him. He was missing in action for half an hour. Tim told me that one has to be able to laugh at these situations and that humor is a great healing medicine. I agree with Tim that a sense of humor is therapeutic especially when it comes to facing physical, intellectual, or emotional afflictions.

"Laughter and tears are both responses to frustration and exhaustion. I myself prefer to laugh, since there is less cleaning up to do afterward."

— Kurt Vonnegut

Tim and I also talk about our love and admiration for our caretakers—in his case, his wife Diane, in mine, my husband, Rich. Both sides are affected and challenged—the one walking through the diagnosis and the loved one walking by their side. It is not easy to completely understand what it's like to be a caretaker of the one afflicted. They want to help, but often don't know exactly how to reach us at the most difficult times. *This is hard.* But when God is in the middle of the situation, and hope is sought after, He sorts out the confusion. Life is puzzling, but God knows how to pick up the pieces.

*　　*　　*

Brain tumors are ugly, and sometimes simply vicious—all life threatening or compromising afflictions are. It is not fair that they get to take a loved one away (with or without warning), challenge health, and shatter lives. My family and I volunteered at a National Brain Tumor Society Walk two and a half years after I became a survivor. As I got ready to go, I had these thoughts in mind: I'm going to take my animosity toward brain tumors and turn it into a fuel to fight them. I'll help where I can, then watch each participant, and think, "*With every step you take, walk with your head held high, with the simple determination that one day soon, we will find a cure and eliminate brain tumors.*"

I am one of the fortunate ones who got to wear a *survivor* t-shirt. The atmosphere at the walk was encouraging, filled with determination, yet painful. Underneath one of the tents, families were making signs to honor loved ones lost. It broke my heart to see families holding signs with pictures and names in memory of people they wished were walking beside them. *Those diagnosed do not want to leave their loved ones behind; those who love them don't want to see them go.* And then I was reminded once again of how blessed I am, to be alive.

Understand—all of us will go away for good someday—some will have warning and others will leave when we least expect it. We can't predict those moments because not one of us is God. "Yet you do not know what your life will be like tomorrow. You are just a vapor that appears for a little while and then vanishes away."[4] Life is precious, life is sweet, life is fragile, and not without challenges. And when it evaporates, it can hurt like crazy. But in Heaven, life won't hurt anymore.

Dear one, if you haven't already let God in—do. He is the only way to get to Heaven.

While at the fundraiser, a young boy around the age of five approached me with his dad. The father was in his forties and told me that he had about six more weeks to live because his brain tumor was aggressive, spreading, and inoperable. He looked down at his son, then right back at me and said, "He is my legacy. I love him."

I held back tears, looked at the father, and whispered, "I am so sorry." The dad responded, "Hey son, say hello to Helo." I got down on my knees to say hello to the boy. He looked at me with a temporary smile that turned into a frown and questioned, "Helo, how do I make the ugly tumor leave my daddy's head?" *I wish that I could've answered that question.*

Saddened, I prayed, *God, hold onto this little boy and his family.* I could hardly speak. I just hugged the young boy and gently whispered, "Keep telling your daddy that you love him." He told me that he did every single day. He just didn't want his daddy to go away. It is hard to see a young father who, barring a miracle, is about to die and leave his son here on earth for good.

I will never forget a heartfelt moment with my dad, days before my brain tumor removal surgery. He put his hands on my shoulders, fastened his eyes on mine, did his best to refrain from crying, and said, "Helo, I wish that I could trade places with you. I am in my seventies now and have lived a full life—you are in your late forties and have so much life yet to live." After everything I endured, I understand how blessed I am to be able to say, "I'm still here, Dad—and I love you."

At one point during the fundraiser, all survivors were called to the stage. Many were in wheelchairs, had speech impediments, had odd gaits, or shook. I looked around and realized that I had it good. Again puzzled, I realized that when God restored me to functionality, it was a complete miracle. My family was not walking around with a photo of me mounted on poster board attached to a stick. No one should ever have to do that. It was massively humbling for me to *still* be alive.

* * *

I sat in a clinic one afternoon, waiting for one of my children. A woman got up, left her husband's side, and approached the table next to me to work on a puzzle of a lighthouse. The image of the lighthouse had already been put together because it was easy; the border had also been finished, the way most people put a puzzle together—easy parts first. This woman worked on the difficult parts of the puzzle, trying to match pieces that were similar in color, composing the dark water and sky. I asked her if she liked working on puzzles. She replied that she was not busy with anything else at that moment—just waiting for her appointment. She was subdued. "Life is puzzling," she interjected. I told her that I pray when life gets hard. She did the same.

She continued to put the puzzle together while telling me that twenty years ago, one month after getting married, she had been diagnosed with breast cancer, and had a double mastectomy. Her husband had stayed by her side, their love had grown, and he is still by her side today. "But sometimes," she said, "*he is grumpy.*" They never were able to conceive children. This was his second marriage, and she was blessed with stepchildren. Two of them loved her; one of them never has.

She was in the office that day for chemotherapy. Cancer was rapidly spreading throughout her body, and she was exhausted. She was determined to fight hard and knew that she could only do so by the grace of God. We concluded that facing death is often a time when people seek God because they realize that life here is temporary; then they frantically ask the "big" questions like whether God and Heaven exist. Sometimes, people seek God when they lose loved ones.

She was thankful that she had asked God into her life decades ago. He made her life complete, and she was not afraid. She had become "older and wiser" and learned that God has a purpose for everything—*because He is wiser than we are.*

We talked about how hard it was to face illness, and she commented that puzzles come in all different shapes and sizes. Some are hard; others are easy. Because she knew and loved God, she understood that Heaven was her final home.

Her husband had been sitting in the waiting room for more than an hour now; her appointment was running late, and he was getting frustrated. She told me that his anger stressed her out, and stress interfered with her healing. I agreed and commented how a patient husband makes a big difference. I promised to pray for both of them.

She excused herself for a moment, saying that she had something to tell her husband. I overheard her telling him, "Helo said that she will pray for us, and you need to start praying for us, too, instead of being grumpy. It interferes with my healing." She came back to me and told me that he said, "I am too grouchy to stop being grumpy." I think he was exasperating her.

I asked her if they liked to walk in parks when it was sunny in Seattle. They had not been on a walk together for a long time, she told me. Then she walked back to her husband and told him, "Helo told me that it is sunny outside and we should go for a walk together." She thanked me for listening to her and for sharing my story. Then she went to her appointment. Her husband stopped me, thanked me for listening to his wife, and told me that they would hold hands and go for a walk together afterwards.

To this day, it still puzzles me why God healed me and does not physically heal everyone—it's a question that only He can answer. But in spite of this, I know that God is still our Healer. His healing does not involve only our physical beings; He also restores our souls. God has the answers to all of the puzzles in our lives because He is God.

God has the power to prevent suffering, but also allows it. He ultimately healed us through the sacrifice of His precious Son, Jesus: "But He was pierced for our transgressions, He was crushed for our iniquities; the punishment that brought us peace was on Him, and by his wounds we are healed."[5] His love is always there for the taking. Ask Him into your heart and you shall receive. God knows how to put the puzzles of our lives together.

Chapter Seventeen

INTENTIONS

If you tell the truth, you don't have to remember anything.

— Mark Twain —

We all go through times of affliction, either because of sin—which none of us are immune from, or because of things beyond our control. To endure these difficulties, we need hope and truth. When we come face to face with these qualities, we are strengthened and encouraged to go on. Our intention is never to fall down, but all of us do, at one time or another.

"For who is God besides the Lord? And who is the Rock except our God? It is God who arms me with strength and keeps my way secure."

— Psalm 18:31–32

I never asked for my journey to involve a brain tumor diagnosis and removal. As difficult as it has been, though, I would not trade it for anything, given all that I have learned.

Rich has completed and filed our taxes with the IRS for decades. He is always diligent and precise and had never thought of hiring an accountant to help him. I had my surgery in January and stayed in the hospital through March. While I was in the hospital, he became completely exhausted. He kept me company constantly and passed some time by working on tax preparation. He thought that he could handle it just as he had in the past, so he filled out the required forms and sent them in. However, a year after I came home, the IRS informed us that Rich had made a significant mistake with our joint tax filing. We met with an accountant who went through our paperwork and corrected the unintentional error. We immediately wrote the check for the fee due and sent it to the IRS together with our accountant's documentation.

The IRS, however, imposed additional fees for "intention to defraud the government." Now, it seems like it would be common sense to know that when someone has a loved one in the hospital on life support, they are under a significant amount of stress. In Rich's situation, this meant that he made some stress-induced mistakes while filing taxes, but he is one determined man.

We negotiated with the IRS for almost a year with the help of our knowledgeable and compassionate accountant. She made it clear to the IRS that Rich had been under significant turmoil while compiling his tax filing because his wife was in a life-threatening position in the hospital. Our accountant truthfully emphasized that Rich had never "intentionally" tried to defraud the government.

We waited for several weeks, only to hear that the IRS rejected this explanation. They said that the fine was accurate and would not be adjusted. We were obviously frustrated because Rich had not done this with intention. Our accountant sent forty pages of documentation to the IRS.

My patience has been tested in many ways. Stress like this does not sit well with me. Paying an unjust fine to the government was like pouring salt into a deep and painful wound. Rules and regulations have their place. No one should be allowed to break the law and get away with it. But our mistake was not intentional. And so we prayed.

At last, the accountant finally had the opportunity to talk "live" with an individual from the IRS. They had all of our unopened documentation on file and finally reviewed the contents. The fine for "intentional attempt to defraud the government" was removed.

The truth won out.

Coinciding with the IRS issue, we spent significant time working with our healthcare provider. My heart goes out to those who do not have health insurance. My total medical bills approached one million dollars. Our insurance company promptly paid for their portion of everything except for the second preparatory embolization procedure. They initially claimed that I had secondary insurance, which I did not. I was a stay-at-home mom and had not worked outside the home for more than two decades. The insurance company questioned why the procedure had been done twice and continually refused a significant payment to my interventional radiologist, who had performed the procedure to protect my life.

Months into this dispute, we submitted complete documentation of the events of my surgery so our remaining medical bills would not be sent to a collection agency. We explained every procedure, drug, piece of equipment and supply, every day spent in the hospital, and every medical staff member necessary. The health insurance company sat on the unopened documentation for more than six months.

Two years after surgery, this situation was still not resolved. We talked about getting legal counsel, but Rich and I had been through enough. *Revisiting this was not fun.* The added stress of countless phone calls with our insurance provider was frustrating. They continually informed us that everything would be paid for, and then it wasn't. Roller coaster rides may be fun in a theme park, but not when it comes to insurance. We continued to be patient and continued to ask God to help us with this confounding mess.

One day, I opened the mail and found a summary of payments on my medical bills. Our insurance company had finally decided to pay for a portion of the second preparatory embolization procedure; they agreed to pay for the anesthesia. I thought, "*You have got to be kidding me. They agree to pay for the need to knock me out, but not for the procedure itself. Who are the people making these decisions?*"

Then I talked with the insurance provider and they asked me to submit proof as to why I needed to have the procedure. I thought, "*Really? Let's see—brain tumors are not supposed to be in someone's head. If a patient is at risk to bleed to death during tumor removal, it sounds like a wise idea to pull out all stops to prevent it."* An in-house MD needed to review my file to determine if the second embolization procedure had been necessary. I thought, *"I wish none of this had been necessary."* Our insurance provider's "prove it to us" attitude added insult to injury. I asked if the in-house MD was a skilled neurosurgeon, because I wanted to make sure that he understood the necessity of the preparatory procedure based upon the credentials of my exceptional neurosurgeon. He was not, so my neurosurgeon agreed to send a letter to him.

Rich managed the situation for me, as he had countless times before. After many more calls and e-mails, the insurance company finally determined to cover not only the anesthesia but also the procedure itself.

Life happens, intentionally or unintentionally. Sometimes things hurt and weigh us down unexpectedly. The situation with the IRS and our medical insurance coverage pushed me to the edge; that wasn't the case for my husband, though, because he is stronger than I am. I needed to listen intentionally to God and to trust Him to provide. I needed to laugh more often, let go of frustration, and move on with patience. That is what finding hope does.

In the big scheme of things, this was small, and didn't matter as much as I had originally thought. I kept thinking, *"When will this be over?—Haven't we been through enough already?"* I have often heard that God will not give us more than we can handle, but I started to question Him, thinking, *"God must think that I am stronger than I am."* God's intention is never that we handle all circumstances on our own. He loves us. We get to hand over our troubles to Him. He wants to walk by our sides through adversity, not for us to "backpack" it all. When we recognize this beautiful characteristic of God, we will be blessed: "Blessed is the one who perseveres under trial because, having stood the test, that person will receive the crown of life, which God has promised to those who love Him."[1]

We all go through times of affliction, as a result of sin, self-induced carelessness, or because things happen to us completely beyond our control. In each of these circumstances, we need to pull hope and truth close to us. These virtues strengthen and grace us with the courage to go on.

Chapter Eighteen

DANCE WITH ME, JESUS

The Lord is my strength and song.

— Exodus 15:2 KJV —

Sometimes trepidation is brutal and real. Fear is the result of lack of trust in the only One who can give complete peace. When we ask God to hold onto us in His arms, He provides comfort in uncomfortable moments: "Peace I leave with you; my peace I give you. I do not give to you as the world gives. Do not let your hearts be troubled and do not be afraid."[1]

Once a year for a total of five years, and then again at year eight, I will go in for a brain MRI. This is a time when Satan dances around in my thoughts and tries to make me afraid. I tell him to back off, and I ask Jesus to dance with me instead.

Right around year two, when I went in for my annual MRI, anxious thoughts consumed me, so I prayed and asked my husband to do likewise. Later, Rich shared with me that a friend at work, Ed, had been a brain tumor-removal survivor for more than a decade. Ed and I set up a time to talk. Peace often comes from talking with someone who has an automatic understanding of our uneasiness. We don't have to explain ourselves because the other understands our fears, and we don't need to justify our feelings; they are simply acknowledged. Ed understood the fear of having to go in for a brain MRI following a tumor removal. Our conversation helped me to feel calm.

We do not always understand God's reasoning behind what He allows us to go through, or why we find ourselves in the position of having to do certain things. His ways are not our ways. We may have the opportunity to help someone else, and in doing so, receive the encouragement that we need.

I walked into Seattle Radiologists, nervous. I had to sit still in the waiting room, but it wasn't easy. I was about to lie down in a machine to see if my brain was tumor free. I was told it likely would be, but I was still worried. Just about anyone who has to go in for something like this would be anxious.

While I sat in the waiting room, I saw a family of five sitting against the wall and told Rich that I felt moved to talk with them. He asked me if I was going to share my story. I didn't know.

I could tell which one of the family members was going in. A young woman in her twenties was clasping the hands of her husband or boyfriend. With her other hand, she was holding on tightly to the hands of her mother, who was holding back tears. The young woman's grandmother sat on the other side of them, obviously concerned.

I walked up and said, "Hi, my name is Helo. Please do not hesitate to ask me to step aside or leave you to your privacy if you want. May I ask which one of you is going in?" The young woman looked up at me and replied, "I am." The entire family looked at me with blank stares, obviously overwhelmed. I asked for the girl's name. She said, "I am 'Claire.'"[2] I told Claire that she would receive excellent care at Seattle Radiologists.

When her family asked me how I knew that, I told them that I'd been here often and that the physicians and technologists were very skilled. I told them that my dad was a medical doctor, that I'd been a pharmaceutical representative, and was quite familiar with the medical environment. I then asked who she was seeing. Her family told me that she was seeing Dr. Raisis.

I stopped and paused.

Dr. Raisis was the excellent physician who had saved my life. I talked with him face to face earlier that day, before I went in for my MRI. I cannot explain in words what it was like to sit in a room with my earthly hero. Looking forward, I can't imagine what it will be like to sit next to our Heavenly Father, who watched over my surgical team, gave my family strength to endure, stayed by my side, and then performed a miracle. "Bless the

Lord, O my soul, and forget not all His benefits: Who forgives all your iniquities, Who heals all your diseases, Who redeems your life from destruction, Who crowns you with loving kindness and with tender mercies."3

I reassured Claire and her family that she was in excellent hands. She asked me how I knew this, so I shared with her my excellent outcome and recovery directed by Dr. Raisis. I did not share the details surrounding my rare extended hospital stay because I did not want to frighten her.

I suggested, "Okay, now when I go into the MRI machine, you pray for me, and when you go in, I'll be praying for you." I did not ask her what her faith was, but I did tell her that there is simplicity to faith. I shared, "We can ask our Maker for peace and help at any moment; at times like this, He is the only One to go to."

It was close to dinnertime, so I suggested to Claire that when she went into the MRI machine to pretend that she was getting ready for a date: "Go into the closet, look through your clothes, and decide what to wear. Choose a restaurant. Imagine waiting to be seated and then finding a table together. Look at the menu and decide what you would like to eat. You aren't hungry right now, are you?"

"Of course not," she countered.

I continued talking and added, "Just walk through your evening, and before you know it, the technologist in the MRI room will lift the lid and say that you are free to go."

The entire family expressed their thankfulness that I had stopped to talk with them. We then all sat around and watched a video on YouTube about cats. Hands were no longer clutched. Nervousness faded. We were all just laughing at the cats that God made—they can be so cute and funny at times. The very people, whom God called upon me to help, reduced my fear and comforted me in return; my anxiety faded, and I went in calmly for my brain MRI.

The technologist gave me earplugs because the machine makes a lot of noise. He strapped my head down to secure it in place and told me to hold my head still. I thought, "*I couldn't move it much if I tried; it's strapped in and the sides surrounding my head are stuffed with gauze.*" I was handed a small ball-like piece of equipment attached to a long chord. The technologist instructed, "Squeeze it if you need to stop." I smiled and thought, "*Humph, can I squeeze it now?*"

Right before the lid of the machine shut over me, I asked God to break me free from the bondage of anxiety, fear, and worry. And He did. "Be anxious for nothing, but in everything by prayer and supplication, with thanksgiving, let your requests be made known to God; and the peace of God, which surpasses all understanding, will guard your hearts and minds through Christ Jesus."[4]

Lying down, I listened to the different beats and sang to myself in cadence with the machine: "Savior, keep me strong; Savior, keep me strong. God, you are my healer; God, you are my healer. I trust you, Jesus; I trust you, Jesus. You make me still when I am restless; You make me still when I am restless. You will never leave my side; You will never leave my side. Hope starts, stays, and lasts with Jesus; Hope starts, stays, and lasts with Jesus. Your grace sets me free; Your grace sets me free. In You my hope is found; In You my hope is found."

I felt like breaking out into a dance, but if I did, the technologist would've told me to stop wiggling my feet. I had to lie completely still or the procedure would have to be repeated. *I did not want to start over.* I was reminded once again: "Be still and know that I am God."[5] I spent more than an hour in the machine, talking with God, and that conversation made it feel like the procedure only lasted fifteen minutes. Through deep dependence on Him, I found peace. He guarded my heart and mind as I danced with Jesus.

Dr. Raisis happened to be in the building that evening, so I didn't have to wait long to get my results. He examined the MRI, came out, and exclaimed that my brain was beautiful! And so, sometimes we go to do things that we may not want to, but God can then use us to help others also in need.

Chapter Nineteen

NOT BY ACCIDENT

To every thing there is a season,
and a time to every purpose under the Heaven.
— Ecclesiastes 3:1 KJV —

One year after starting to drive again, I got rear-ended in my car by a young man. I was yielding to oncoming traffic in a roundabout. I stopped, then slowly inched forward to get a better view of the vehicles in the roundabout. Instead of taking his turn to yield, the driver behind me punched the gas pedal and rear-ended me. We both got out and looked at each other. He hesitated, "You must be really angry with me."

I replied, "I am not 'really angry' with you, but I am not happy with what just happened here." He wanted to leave the scene, simply giving me his phone number. He looked as though he was thinking, "*My dad is going to kill me!*"

If this had happened prior to my near-Heaven experience, I would have gotten pretty ticked, but things are different now. I told him that I was not furious, but he was in trouble, and could not leave the scene. I called the police, then we both pulled our cars off to the side of the road.

I had been on my way to pick up my son, Jordan, from school. I thought, "*How am I supposed to get him now?*" I texted him first, to let him know about the accident, and told him to stay at the library. Then I texted my husband and our two other children. They prayed for me. I texted my dad next, and he said to call him after I was done with the police officers, because we needed to discuss a possible neck injury. *It hurt.*

The young man asked, "Why aren't you mad? If I were in your shoes I would be livid."

I scolded, "Well, my neck hurts, my car has been dented, your car hood is crushed, my son is waiting to be picked up, and I have a lot to do today. But I'm not mad, because you and I are alive."

He looked at me, confused, and said, "Huh?"

I shared an abbreviated version of my story.

He simply replied, "Wow."

I don't know what he thought of God's promises. He was understandably preoccupied with the trouble that he was in at the moment.

My neck hurt, and the officers asked me if I wanted to file an injury report right away. An ambulance would come immediately, I'd be evaluated, strapped to a gurney with a neck brace, and taken to the nearest emergency room. My neck hurt, but I had no interest whatsoever in going to a hospital, because I had been there, done that. I likely would sit for hours in the ER while I waited to be examined. I told the two police officers that I did not want to go. *Not today.*

They noted my neck pain on the police report, listened to both versions of the accident, and asked more questions. My brake lights were checked and then the two officers sent me on my way. I called my husband and dad on my way to get my son. As I left, the young man was corralled by the two officers, because I had stated earlier that he had wanted to flee the scene. He received a ticket.

Later, my son and I stopped for anti-inflammatory medication, per doctor's orders. Then I applied ice at home, was examined by my dad, took pain medications, and moved my neck continually. Later, I'd do physical therapy for several weeks and make countless phone calls with insurance. *It's no fun getting rear-ended.*

I told Jordan about my accident that afternoon. He asked if I was okay, and I assured him that I was fine. He said, "If I just rear-ended someone, I would be mad at myself, and need time to cool down." Then he smiled and added, "I might ask the officer to put me in jail for just one night so that I could avoid the immediate wrath of my parents." I used this as an opportunity to implement Driving 101 because Jordan was learning how to drive at the time. Smiling, I explained, "When a car in front of you inches up toward a yield sign, it does not mean—accelerate."

I took my car to a collision repair company and parked my car in a wheelchair spot. The receptionist handed me paperwork to fill out. I sat down, put my keys and purse on the table, and started filling out the necessary documents. A cute little boy learning how to walk waddled over to me and started to fiddle around with my paperwork. I found it entertaining; he was having fun while making a mess. The boy's father did not find it funny and apologized. I smiled and told him to enjoy his child to the fullest every day because he would grow up in a hurry. He replied, "Yeah, I try, but sometimes I get irritated with him."

I understood.

The dad asked me how old my kids were, and I told him they were twenty-one, seventeen, and fourteen. He asked me if I loved them more now than I had when they were little. "Absolutely!" I exclaimed, "I've gotten to know them better every day."

He said, "It does not really feel that way right now. My son is only fourteen months old, and I've got a long way to go." I told him that I used to feel that way, until I had come close to dying two years before. He asked me "How? You look healthy and too young to have three kids at your children's ages." I shared the outline of my journey, and he said, "Amazing story, thank you for sharing. Oops, got to go—my little one is trying to take off." I thought, "*He hasn't seen anything yet. Wait until his son is a teenager.*" I told him to take care, and finished my paperwork.

Then a woman close to my age sat down next to me. She told me that she had overheard my conversation and hoped that I'd be willing to talk with her. "No problem," I said. She had been rear-ended a couple of days prior. I agreed with her that it was no fun. She wanted to go deeper than that in our conversation, though. She was panicking because she was going in for a brain and spinal MRI the very next day. I asked her if she minded sharing her story.

She had gotten tired of telling others why or when she was going in, because they either didn't know what to say or asked her insensitive questions, but she felt comfortable talking to me. Her eyes welled up with tears. She was in her late forties and had multiple sclerosis (MS). Her neurologist had increased her MRI studies to once every three months, instead of every six. *The MS had progressed.* She had been going in for the past four years and believed that the MS had contibuted to her increasing anxiety about having MRIs.

Claustrophobia set in. She was terrified of the lid closing down on her. If she tried to calm down, the very thing that she was trying to relax about came to the forefront of her mind and she panicked. I explained that I'd gone through my share of MRIs and understood the anxiety. I shared with her how I "rapped" to the MRI machine cadence while inside of it. I told her that when the technologist told me not to move my head, I thought, *"Are you kidding me? My head is strapped down. How could I move it, even if I wanted to?"*

It felt like forced potential claustrophobia. A speaker would come on and the technologist would calmly say, "Now it will be three and a half minutes," and the beat would change. Then the speaker would come on again and the technologist would say, "Now it will be five minutes," and so on. I explained my "Dance with Jesus" approach to her and told her that it felt like the MRI session lasted fifteen minutes rather than an hour or more.

She felt encouraged, smiled, and said, "I'll try your approach tomorrow." She was thankful that we had talked, and appreciated our conversation. We each picked up our paperwork and walked out to our cars. Then I thought, *"Okay, God, maybe this is why I got rear-ended. Maybe this is why she did also."*

* * *

After getting the collision repair assessment report, I called my assigned insurance agent. She was unavailable, so another agent helped me instead. She pulled up my claim file, needing to ask me several questions: How was my neck? What medical attention had I sought or received? What medications had I taken?

Then I became quiet.

She asked, "Are you all right?"

I replied, "I've been on a huge number of medications, seen an ample number of physicians over the past couple of years and don't like talking about the details.

"Doctors can be helpful."

"Yeah, the police offered to send me to the emergency room via an ambulance, but I'm 'doctored out.'"

"Can I ask you why you feel that way?"

"Sure."

I hesitated, then I spoke up and stated, "Brain tumor removals aren't fun and I learned all about that the hard way, but God stayed with me."

"What?"

I told her more. Then I heard nothing on the other end of the line. Complete silence.

"Are you still there?" I asked.

After a few moments, she told me, "You are beautiful, Helo. I needed to talk with someone just like you today. We have over a hundred representatives taking calls. To think that I took your call because the assigned representative on your case was on another line is incredible. It was meant to be!"

Silence again.

I asked, "Are you all right?"

"I'm okay—but I lost my dad to a brain tumor three years ago."

Goosebumps ran up and down my arms. I wished that we were talking in person rather than over the phone.

"First off, I am so sorry that you lost your dad."

She thanked me. A few people had reminded her that it had been three years, the implication being that it was time to get over her loss. I told her that three years can feel like three weeks or three months when you have lost a loved one; everyone deals with the pain at a different pace. Those who die before us take a precious part of us away. The pain never completely vanishes but softens and becomes a reminder of how much we loved those we lost.

I did not want to make her cry in front of her peers at work. She didn't mind talking to me about her father and commented that I was amazing. Humbled at the response, I replied, "God is the amazing One."

She agreed. We talked for several more minutes, and she told me all that she loved about her dad. She knew where he was now because he loved God, and that comforted her.

I suggested that she should get back to work, but she preferred to continue talking, because she found our conversation reassuring, and an answer to prayer. She was blessed by talking with someone who understood what a brain tumor can do to a family. I was blessed by the reminder of how much God loves us and what He has promised us in Heaven. I told her to reflect upon all of the things that she loved about her dad, to rest in knowing where he is today, and reminded her that one day she would see him again. Neither one of us wanted to get off the phone, but we both understood God's purpose behind our conversation, and then said our "good-byes."

"For you, Lord, have delivered me from death, my eyes from tears, my feet from stumbling, that I may walk before the Lord in the land of the living."[1] We are all going to die someday; some will inevitably leave before us, and it will hurt. We all have or will face struggles. Not one of us can avoid the inevitable. God knows all of life's occurrences in advance, they are not accidental, rather He allows them for His intended purpose. Often, He is simply waiting for us to say, "God, I just realized that you stay by my side all of the time, even when life gets hard. Now, I need to stop and look for your affection." God alone can make life beautiful, even through the darkness of affliction, because He loves us with intention—never by accident.

Chapter Twenty

MORE THAN A SURVIVOR

*But we have this treasure in jars of clay to show
that this all-surpassing power is
from God and not from us.*

— 2 Corinthians 4:7 —

God, the Master Potter, molded me through suffering. He taught me about His love and empowered me to endure. *He is amazing.* Through an intimidating and unimaginable trial, I saw His unique love. In the middle of a storm, we may not always see God's reasons for allowing that pain, yet He can strengthen and mold us like clay. He will always be by our side, and His presence makes us new.

In hindsight, I see why God has allowed certain trials in my life. Other trials I do not yet understand, and won't until I meet Him face to face. God alone has perfect wisdom. He has a purpose for everything. I have learned to fight fear that prevents me from pursuing God's love and protection. "We are afflicted in every way, but not crushed; perplexed, but not driven to despair."[1] God goes before us in our battles and comforts us in our despairs.

I am a survivor, who recognized the One, who never left my side— *God.* He blessed me with authentic courage, and I discovered where true hope is found. I want to encourage others to hold on, and never give up. When you stumble into feelings of defeat, do not stay there. *Hold onto God.* He has been holding onto you all along; you just may not know it yet.

I learned quickly that being a survivor is just the start of a challenging journey. I survived physical and emotional trauma. My brain tumor frightened me in a very real way, and I don't know all of the reasons why God allowed it, but I am starting to understand some of them. I also don't know why He chose to keep me alive, but He did. And that is not the end of this story. He miraculously healed me, and I am determined to tell others about it, revealing hope and courage.

It is difficult to relive my story every time I share it, but if I am quiet about what only God can do, then I would not be rising to the challenge He put before me. I never asked for any of this, and I don't want pity. As Helen Keller said, "Self pity is our worst enemy and if we yield to it, we can never do anything wise in this world." I am a fighter, a sinner, a survivor, and a cherished child of God who needs His love more than anything else. *I know that you need His love too—I haven't met anyone who doesn't, but I've met plenty who think they don't.*

God did something big for me, and I will not wrap myself in survival mode. I am not a survivor in a cage. Rather, I will stand and share His glorious ability to make every one of us whole. I will never be the same, and I can't return to the way life once was. Those who learn how much their Maker loves them will never be the same.

Faith in Him can restore us and make us better than we can believe ourselves to be. I will not define myself merely a disabled person, because "I can do all things through Christ who strengthens me."[2] God gave me a story and made me a survivor; He went before me into battle. "The Lord is my strength and my shield; My heart trusted in Him, and I am helped; Therefore my heart greatly rejoices, And with my song I will praise Him."[3]

I want to be whole, not just survive.

I used to cry a lot about my struggles and ask, *"God, why me?"* Then God told me to challenge my limitations. He didn't always take them away from me. He watched and encouraged me to get up by myself on purpose. At times I screamed, "Pick me up right now, God!" But He didn't, and that response made me strong, so now I am a more than a survivor. *Steadfast, transparent, and a humble faith in God makes me complete.* I used to be a patient who needed constant help, but now I get to take care of, and sometimes inspire others.

January 31, 2013—that was the second anniversary of my admission to the hospital to begin preparation for my brain tumor removal. I reflected on what God had pulled me through. January 31, 2013, was also the day on which my mom had eye surgery. Over the course of a year, she had been through five surgeries to repair a detached retina. The first one, an emergency procedure to prevent blindness, had taken place in Prague while she and my dad were on vacation. I told both my mom and dad that this time, I wanted to be there for them.

It was time to get ready to go to the hospital to see my mom. I showered and washed my hair with ease before dressing quickly without any help. I attended to my boys; took care of the dogs; made necessary phone calls; grabbed my cell phone, purse, and keys; and jetted out the door. Then a flashback hit. Once, I had left the boys alone for what I had thought would be six days but it turned into eight weeks. I had prepared the home as much as possible before leaving for the hospital that time, but this time it was easier and different. I knew that after my mom's surgery, I'd return home.

Once in my car, I realized that I had forgotten something. I went back into the house and saw that the back door was open. Thankfully, I closed the door. We had recently gotten our puppy, Buttons. Several days prior, Buttons had run away because the back door had been left open. We had been scared for her safety, but then she had come back home, wet and muddy. We had hugged her even though she was a complete mess! In a minuscule way, embracing our muddy puppy reminded me of how much God loves us in the midst of our messes, and is joyful when we are not longer lost, but found.

While driving to see my parents, I had another flashback. I remembered what it was like to drive to the hospital for my surgery: I had been shaking, huddled in a warm blanket. I'd clasped my brave husband's right hand as he had driven with his left. But this hospital visit was different. I parked in a wheelchair spot and walked through the door of the clinic. Anxious to join my parents, I looked for my dad in the waiting room.

Concern distorted the faces of families, spouses, and patients in the waiting room. I prayed for them. Then my dad opened the door from the surgical unit and said, "Helo, thank you for coming." I hugged him, and we went back to see my mom. I held her hand, kissed her forehead, and said, "Everything is going to be okay."

It was surreal. I was now a miraculous survivor, not a patient, sitting in a pre-operative room with medical equipment, emergency buttons, a crash cart, a blanket warmer, and nurses in blue surgical clothing. I listened to the beeping and swishing noise of machines. My mom got on the pre-op bed to be moved into surgery. She had on a blue surgery cap and gown, and a blue blood pressure cuff that was continually tightening and relaxing. There were markings on her forehead, an IV drip, and oxygen tubes going into her nose. She didn't want to have anything put up her nose, and I couldn't blame her; I hated having the feeding tube up my nose and had tried to yank it out. I looked at her and smiled, saying, "You are stubborn like me. I know exactly where I got it from."

She replied, "I am done!" and I had another flashback. I used to say the same thing during inpatient rehabilitation.

A nurse, Deanne, visited with us. My parents told her that I'd recently been through a hard time, and she asked about it. I explained that I was a brain tumor survivor. Both Deanne's brother and a close girlfriend had gone through recent brain tumor removals. The friend was not doing well because the tumor was cancerous, and she had lost a lot of weight during chemotherapy. Deanne's brother had been diagnosed with a brain tumor after having a massive seizure one day. I prayed for them.

My parents and I waited in the pre-op room for quite a while. I watched my dad sit by his wife, my precious mom. He is an amazing husband and had been a caring doctor. I had another flashback. My dad stayed by my mom's side, and my husband had done the same thing for me.

Mom became frustrated as we waited. She wanted to go get a cup of coffee; she loved Starbucks. Dad informed her that the surgery would then be postponed. "Now, that's an idea! Coffee could be a way to get out of this?" she asked. I told Mom that she was being stubborn. Dad then asked if she thought he was ever stubborn.

I interrupted, joking, "Why be stubborn when no one is telling you what to do?" We got a chuckle out of that.

We continued to wait, and Dad shared a story. Long ago, as a medical student, he had taken an IV bag from the hospital and watered our Christmas tree with it. Deanne asked him if he had been able to refill the bag with water and reuse it. He smiled and answered, "Yes." I smiled too and realized that I needed to set up a date with him to hear more of these mischievous stories.

Another nurse came in and looked at Mom's wristband. She confirmed Mom's date of birth and asked her if the left eye was the one being repaired. Mom replied, "The doc better operate on the right one—the left." The nurse then checked if Mom had any allergies and asked her a host of other questions. Mom was almost ready to be taken back; Dad told her that she was one step closer to being done and ready to go home.

The surgeon came out to talk with us. My mom wanted to get started and did not want to hear anything at all from the doctors as they moved her into the operating room. The surgeon asked her, "Anything to drink? Any cough? Any difficulty breathing? Do you have any questions for me?"

Her reply to every question was a resounding, "No!"

Then he asked her, "Are you ready to go in?"

She exclaimed, "Yes."

"Okay, then let me go back and get all our ducks in a row. Then we will get started," the surgeon teased.

Mom snickered and quipped, "It's time for the docs to get in a row, not the ducks." God has gifted her with a sense of humor to get through difficult moments.

Hugs and kisses led to another flashback: my family had done the same for me.

My mom was under excellent care. Dad and I had lunch together, and I asked if he was doing okay. He mentioned that this had been hardest for

Mom. Six eye surgeries were far too many. She hadn't been able to see through her left eye for over a year now. She sometimes shut down and did not want to talk about it. Sometimes, my dad covered one of his eyes for a while to see what it was like for Mom; even then, he couldn't truly understand. I had another flashback: Sometimes I had told Rich that I wished he could walk in my shoes for only half an hour to understand how I now felt.

My mom sometimes coped by staying frustrated instead of just moving on with her "disability" of impaired vision. She didn't want us to ask her how she was doing daily, and I understood that. When I'd come home, I sometimes found myself feeling down and did not want to explain why.

The surgeon came out of the operating room to say that all had gone well with Mom's surgery and that she was waking up. We went back to give her a hug. I high-fived her and had a flashback to the day when I had weakly waved to her in the ICU. On this day, I was happy to see my mom and content to know that she was going to be okay. Then I went home.

January 31, 2013, was my two-year anniversary of the beginning of brain tumor removal. I got to tell my children, "Good night, I love you." It's a beautiful thing to be able to say. I had the joy of snuggling with my husband and letting him know how much I love him. We got to pray together, asking for many more anniversaries. We'll appreciate every one of them that God gifts us with and thank Him for who He is.

Disabilities can result in enormous physical and emotional loss. I now have the strength to reach out to those who are disabled, emotionally struggling, challenged with affliction, and working hard to overcome life-altering obstacles. After hearing my story, a young man once told me, "Surviving an experience like that should now make every day a great one."

Then God said to me, "Helo, there is more to this than simply becoming a survivor."

It is exciting to share how amazing God's love is. I know that He is not finished with me yet. He is not finished with you, either. He stayed by my side over and over again. When you intentionally call Him to your side, you will transparently see that He will do the same for you. He is closer to you than you might think, "For I am convinced that neither death nor life, neither angels nor demons, neither the present nor the future, nor any powers, neither height nor depth, nor anything else in all creation, will be able to separate us from the love of God that is in Christ Jesus our Lord."4

*   *   *

Becoming more than a survivor means that I now get to support others. I received a call from my husband one morning after he went to the lab to receive IV antibiotics. "What for?" I asked. His dermatologist had just informed him that he had a dangerous scalp infection. Later, he learned that she was fearful of Hodgkin's lymphoma because his lymph nodes were so swollen. Thankfully, that was not the case.

I went to the lab. As I walked back to see Rich, I could tell that people received chemotherapy there, and so I prayed for them. When I opened the curtain and saw my husband sitting there, it felt like another bad dream. He was attached to an IV—I clung to his hand, which reassured both of us. We sat there for only one hour, but it felt longer. A thought struck me: *"My husband sat by me for weeks, and now I get to sit by his side and help him in his time of need. Thank you, God."*

*   *   *

One day more than a year after surgery, I returned to Dick's Drive-In with my son Jordan. This was the place where I'd gotten to eat a lunch out while hospitalized, as part of my physical therapy, compliments of the rehabilitation unit. My return brought back memories of that adventure. Unlike the last time, this time was simple. Jordan and I ordered burgers and fries and sat together in the car. It's hard to explain just how much I enjoyed this moment with my son. God had helped me in a perilous time of need. I can never match His grace, and there is no guarantee that He will rescue me in the way that I want, every time when I am in trouble, but I will pay attention to His whispers reminding me of the importance of helping those in need: "Blessed is he who considers the poor; The Lord will deliver him in time of trouble."[5]

Just as we were about to leave, I saw a homeless man grabbing used burger sacks out of the garbage. No one should have to eat this way. He sat behind the back of the building and began eating his lunch consisting of remnants from another. *I was taken aback.* I quickly handed my son cash and told him to get this gentleman a freshly made burger and fries. Jordan bought the lunch and handed it to this hungry man, who smiled from ear to ear as he opened the bag. He did not savor it; he scarfed it down. Watching him, reminded me of how much all of us are in need to one degree or another.

God helped me to fight a harrowing battle. He told me, "Beloved, it is not yet time for you to come home, and now you are more than a survivor. Until the day that you return to stay for eternity, please continue to share with others how much I love and cherish them." I am more than a survivor. I am more than a conqueror—because when Jesus walked me through the midst of suffering, He showed me something more: Hope can rise and carry us out of the chains of affliction. And to that I say, "Amen."

Chapter Twenty-One

HOPE FOUND

The most precious hope is found in the beautiful One who loved and loves us, saved and saves us.

— Helo —

Brought to a complete stop, I was frail and motionless. Then God said, "I promise you will enter the Kingdom of Heaven someday, just not yet, my cherished child." I woke up to the exhausting challenge of learning how to do just about everything over again. Walking upright was once something that I thought I'd never be able to do on my own. But now I can, both outwardly and inwardly. God loved me first, never quit on me, and now I will strive to always love Him in return.

I'm not the same as I was before my brain tumor removal and recovery. And had it not been discovered and removed with God's timing—I wouldn't be here today. The challenge of regaining my "new normal" has transfomed my soul in an incredible way. I now know with transparency the One who made and loves me—and you. He loves every one of us right down to the very last detail, like no one else can. I'll never take life for granted again. Or at least now I am better at trying not to.

I have been blessed by the assurance that faith grows during trials, and I discovered hope with His help. The most difficult parts of our lives, those that tear us to the core, can also be the most valuable because they can lead us to God. He never promised us that we wouldn't face affliction; He simply promised that He is with us. When we call God to our side with our heartfelt wishes, we'll see the evidence of His love, protection, sustenance, and encouragement. We'll recognize that He has always loved us. We have the honor of getting to know our amazing Maker. I don't know how I could get through my day without Him. God completes me—and He can complete you. I had days when I didn't know when, or if I would return home to be a wife, mom, daughter, sister, and friend. This scared me.

My life has been touched by a series of miracles. To say that I'm humbled is an understatement. *"God, I don't know why you allowed my journey, but I trust you to love me and reveal the purpose behind it all. You alone can pull the beauty out of the ashes of a difficult situation."* God did not, and will never back down from me—or from you—after you ask Him to draw near. I can't remain silent about what He's done for me, or all that He's done for you. As Martin Luther King, Jr. once said, "Our lives begin to end the day we become silent about the things that matter."

I'm continually led by God to let others know that no matter what you have experienced or will experience, God can pull you through. He *adores* you. When something difficult happens and God doesn't "fix it" right away, or at all, it doesn't mean that He doesn't love you; He's simply molding you and knows when to release you from your suffering.

"When you pass through the waters, I will be with you; And through the rivers, they shall not overflow you. When you walk through fire, you shall not be burned, nor shall the flame scorch you. For I am the Lord your God..."
— Isaiah 43:2-3 NKJV

Everlasting hope is found when we finally stop, and listen to the One who loves us, as He says, "Child, I can help you carry your burdens, if you let me." I learned to let go and let God. And He stayed beside me, sustaining me through a tough journey. Don't wander away from Him—it'll only make your life harder. When we wander away from God instead of towards Him, it makes way for fear composed by the enemy. Then we ponder defeat before the heat of the battle begins. Hope found in God erases premature defeat, and nourishes the strength to endure the difficulty placed before us. Hope found in the One who loves us is hope found at its best and unleashes a vibrant faith.

Hope is available for all. Joy can be found even when we don't think so: "In all this you greatly rejoice, though now for a little while you may have had to suffer grief in all kinds of trials. These have come so that the proven genuineness of your faith—of greater worth than gold, which perishes even though refined by fire—may result in praise, glory and honor when Jesus Christ is revealed."[1] God makes beauty from ashes; trials build genuine faith. We can rise from struggles when we ask God to be the leader of our battles. This is strength and comfort at its finest. Only He has the capacity to rescue us from the captivity of adversity and to empower us to authentically appreciate hope. If we refuse to seek God with faith, we are neglecting the One who does not abandon us.

He breathes Heavenly hope into our hearts and holds us together. God will make you new if you let Him. I believe that He uses hopeless situations to show us the promise of security and everlasting life, which lie only in Him. He mends broken hearts, gives courage, and heals fractured lives. Fear, shame, and discouragement are diminished or erased, and we are made new. Peace, redemption, courage, determination, resilience, and faith take over. In Him, hope is found.

"We must accept finite disappointment but never lose infinite hope."

— Martin Luther King, Jr.

I saw this over and over again in my journey. I was tired and worn, and sometimes gave up. I felt overwhelmed and showered with affliction. At times, the only prayer I had the strength to whisper was, "God help me." But that was enough. He listens to every single request we have. Hope in Jesus' promise is enough: "Then you would trust, because there is hope; And you would look around and rest securely."[2]

On occasion, people will listen to, or read about a miracle, and they may be moved and changed. At other times, they might think, "*Well, it's great that you made it. The story indicates that there is a God, but where is the rest of the proof that He exists?"* Winston Churchill once wrote, "Men occasionally stumble over the truth, but most of them pick themselves up and hurry off as if nothing had happened." Many ask if God really exists.

"A heathen philosopher once asked a Christian, 'Where is God?' The Christian answered, 'Let me first ask you, Where is He not?'"

— Aaron Arrosmith

Proof is everywhere. Look around you. Those who don't see Him are blind, metaphorically. When we open our eyes unto the Lord, it is mind-blowing to see Him for who He truly is. *Dear one, do not miss out on His love.* Everything that makes up the earth and the universe—the humans that inhabit it, the nature that surrounds us—displays proof that God is real. Creation, in and of itself, is miraculous.

Look at a loved one or a child. I cherish watching my children because God made them. They can play, laugh and dance, keep me company, irritate me, shake my emotions, encourage me with hugs and words, demonstrate artistic skill, show brilliance, breathe, laugh, run, walk, and cry. They achieve goals and tasks, make mistakes, and learn. They're miraculous and I adore them. God loves them even more. Now *that* is one incredible love.

I like to sit outside when it's dark and the sky is clear. I do this often on my front steps, especially after a long day. I look up at the bright stars sparkling in an expansive sky and know that God made them. They're a true reminder that God's light is ever present—even in our dark times. During the day, I like to look up at the clouds moving and watch the sun shining through. I love seeing different images within the clouds, like a bird, a flower, cotton candy, a tree, or an angel. Then I think, *"God made the sky and now I'm having fun with His creation."* I can only imagine how much fun our Maker had when he created it.

Go for a walk in the park or on a beach, listen to what God made. The birds sing, the wind whispers through the leaves, and the waves crash on the shore. Look around you and then up. God understands the doubt that you may have, so He created evidence and then placed it all around us. Question no more His existence and unfailing love.

With faith in our Maker, life will never be the same; it'll be beautiful. Faith will allow us to understand what it means to be protected by His tender watch during times of trouble. It also shows us *who* to praise when life is good. The Bible says, "Therefore we do not lose heart, but though our outer man is decaying, yet our inner man is being renewed day by day. For momentary, light affliction is producing for us an eternal weight of glory far beyond all comparison."[3] *God loves and guards.*

One day, I sat outside on our back patio and heard birds chirping from a nest hidden in some ivy. A mother was feeding her young, and a father was keeping protective watch. She flew back and forth to gather food, and he never left his post. As I watched these birds interact, I thought, "*Who on earth could watch this, as intensely as I am now, and think there is no God? And the God who made them loves us even more.*" The Bible tells us, "Look at the birds of the air; they do not sow or reap or store away in barns, and yet your heavenly Father feeds them. Are you not much more valuable than they?"[4]

God is real. He was real yesterday, He is real today, and He will be real tomorrow. His love is eternal—backwards and forwards, up and down, and side to side—but sometimes, we're too self-absorbed to recognize Him. Perhaps we surmise that He isn't there, think that we're invincible and don't need Him, or figure that life is as good as it's going to get. Friend, this isn't Heaven. If you keep thinking that it is, then this may be the closest that you'll ever get to it. If instead, you recognize that this isn't Heaven, then put your faith in the One who created our eternal Kingdom, and ask for forgiveness of sin.

> "*To enter Heaven is to become more human than you ever succeeded in being on earth; to enter hell, is to be banished from humanity.*"
>
> — C. S. Lewis, The Problem of Pain

Oftentimes, some of us think we know Him as much as we need too. Others of us may allow Him into certain parts of our lives. Then there are those of us who choose to leave Him completely out. It hurts God when we don't reciprocate His affection; but ultimately, choosing to reject Him will hurt us eternally.

Don't miss out on seeing God for who He really is. It's truly a blessing to recognize Him—and then get to know Him. When this happens, we get to see how much He loves us, and experience His buffering from burdens or afflictions, because He holds onto us to make us brave. And the "good life", we thought we had, becomes more beautiful than before. "Then you will know the truth, and the truth will set you free."[5] Knowing God makes life complete. The Almighty cannot be minimized into words on paper, but words *can* introduce who He is, and what He alone can do.

GOD IS AND DOES

God loves with perfection; therefore, His compassion is set apart from all others.

God is the Creator, which proves that He is real.

God is the truth, which means that He washes out lies.

God is infinite and therefore, everlasting.

God is jealous for our affections, which means that He boldly cares.

God is patient, therefore He is willing to wait for us.

God is faithful, so His promises are always fulfilled.

God removes fear, and therefore, quenches doubt.

God gives us strength, which makes Him our sustenance.

God understands our hearts; therefore, He knows us better than anyone else does.

God is our fortress, which means that He is our strong tower of protection.

God is holy, so He is set apart from all created beings.

God is pure; therefore, He never thinks or acts in evil ways.

God infinitely understands, which means that He demonstrates perfect knowledge.

God gives us grace; therefore, He is everything we need.

God commanded the Word to be written, making Him the instructor of our faith.

God heals brokeness and, therefore, restores hearts.

God softens discouragement and, therefore, helps us find hope.

God sacrificed his Son for our sins, which makes Jesus our Redeemer.

God created Heaven, so He is the designer of eternity.

God is amazing, which makes those who see Him stand in awe.

God hears our every whisper; therefore, He is the one to lift up prayers to.

God created voices to sing; therefore, He is to be worshipped.

God's love is precious; therefore, loving Him makes life complete.

— Helo

I've learned a lot about who God is throughout my lifetime. When I first met Him I was around six or seven years old, sitting in church, where I got to use crayons to color in cartoon-like pictures of Jesus with lambs. I got to drink sweet juice poured into a paper filled cup, and enjoy cookies. I loved snacks. I'd try to go back for more but my mom would say, "That's enough, Helo."

I remember singing "Jesus Loves Me." I recently found the song again. I didn't remember all of the verses. But when I look at it today, I see what God had yet to teach me. I am His "child" no matter how old I get. Making it through life's challenges, and finally learning that it's easier to walk with Him than without Him, taught me that, in Him alone, true hope is found. It's wonderful to be caught up in His love. And so, He's going to keep teaching me here, until I leave for good and rest in Heaven.

Jesus Loves Me

Verse 1
Jesus loves me! this I know,
For the Bible tells me so.
Little ones to Him belong;
They are weak, but He is strong.

Chorus
Yes, Jesus loves me!
Yes, Jesus loves me!
Yes, Jesus loves me!
The Bible tells me so.

Verse 2
Jesus loves me! this I know,
As He loved so long ago,
Taking children on His knee,
Saying, "Let them come to Me."

Verse 3
Jesus loves me! He who died,
Heaven's gate to open wide.
He will wash away my sin,
Let His little child come in.

Verse 4
Jesus loves me still today,
Walking with me on my way.

He's prepared a home for me,
And someday His face I'll see.

— Lyrics by Anna B. Warner, Verses 2 and 4
by David R. McGuire[6]

Some might get to this final chapter of this book and say, *"Great, Helo, so you and your family experienced this miracle, but listen to what I'm going through?"* You might then go on to explain with one or more of the following: I feel helpless, I'm unemployed, my loved one has cancer, I'm facing addiction, I feel trapped in my body, I'm a widow, my child committed suicide, I'm disabled, I lost my home, I just got diagnosed with something difficult, I've no money for food, I'm depressed and alone, I'm suffering. It would not surprise me if you then said, *"Where's God if I can't see Him? It feels like He abandoned me."*

I haven't walked in the exact same shoes that you have—*no two people ever do.* But I do know the One who knows how to walk by your side and equip you to be brave. God doesn't abandon us. He listens. He's in control. And everything that takes place under Heaven has a purpose.

A Time for Everything

For everything there is a season,
    a time for every activity under Heaven.
A time to be born and a time to die.
    A time to plant and a time to harvest.
A time to kill and a time to heal.
    A time to tear down and a time to build up.
A time to cry and a time to laugh.
    A time to grieve and a time to dance.
A time to scatter stones and a time to gather stones.
    A time to embrace and a time to turn away.

A time to search and a time to quit searching.
A time to keep and a time to throw away.
A time to tear and a time to mend.
A time to be quiet and a time to speak.
A time to love and a time to hate.
A time for war and a time for peace.

— Ecclesiastes 3:1-8 NLT

Raw emotions of "Why this? Why now? Why me?" are a normal part of the human condition. Although understandable, the weight of questioning and groveling in self pity can pull you under the wrong authority. It's that ugly enemy rearing his presence again. He's mean...and a liar. Don't let the Devil abuse you and delight in your frustration during these moments of not seeking the protection and love of God. Instead, in the middle of chaos, find hope—and you'll see that it's the reflection of Jesus' love. "And the God of all grace, who called you to his eternal glory in Christ, after you have suffered a little while, will himself restore you and make you strong, firm and steadfast."[7]

Every single one of us has a story to tell. We live in a fragile world where everyone has faced, or will face tribulation to one degree or another. Some of us are outspoken, some of us choose to be quiet. "When you struggle, if you sin, or if you think that you can live life completely on your own, all the more reason to get to know Him. For some of us it will be for the first time, for others it will entail a renewed commitment to immerse ourselves in His love. Find hope in God—this is when His love gets real. Dear friend, my simple hope *and* prayer for you is this: that you will find assurance in knowing that when you choose to love Him back, life becomes complete."

I learned to move forward by seeing that God goes before me. My trials are an opportunity to find joy through faith and endurance. "Consider it all joy, my brethren, when you encounter various trials, knowing that the testing of your faith produces endurance. And let endurance have its per-

208

fect result, so that you may be perfect and complete, lacking in nothing."[8]

We all go through trials. It's unrealistic to think that any of us will live a problem-free life or that we can make it void of burdens. *Life here is hard.* We will all encounter obstacles, adversities, and afflictions. We can't jump over or around them, and we cannot hide from them. We have to walk through them and by God's grace we can be brave. He knows how to equip us.

The key to dealing with trials is to ask God in. When we ask Jesus into our hearts we discover something beyond our trials. We find that God has beautiful promises for us, forgiveness of sins, hope in all circumstances, a meaningful life, and the promise of Heaven, where we will no longer experience suffering, pain, or sin.

Many of us make excuses as to why we don't need God, but all of us *do* need him. *Don't overlook God.* Oliver Wendell Holmes once wrote, "The greatest act of faith is when a man understands that he is not God." God is our ultimate judge, no one else. Sometimes we judge others because it's easier to deflect and locate their faults rather than look at our own. Some of us may think that we're too good for God, that we don't need Him, or *maybe even that we aren't good enough for Him.* I've struggled with that last option many times. Then I have this conversation:

"God, why do you love me?"

Because I am love.[9]

"God, when do you love me?"

Always.

"How do You love me?"

With grace, patience, and forgiveness.

"God, am I good enough for you?'

My precious child, you don't need to be.

"Why?"

Because I love you so much that I gave my only Son, and He took upon his shoulders the afflictions and sins of this world.

"God, when will I get to see You?"

After you choose to believe in Me.

"Then I will know You here, and in Heaven?"

Yes, then you will know Me here, and in Heaven.

"I love you, God."

He always replies, *I loved you yesterday, I love you today, and I will love you tomorrow.*

Then I can't seem to get enough of Him—I *want* to spend more time with Him, and life becomes so *beautiful* when I do. God knows our weaknesses, and doubts, and loves us in spite of them. Through Jesus alone, we are seen as perfect in the eyes of God. *My hope starts, stays, and never leaves when I find it in Jesus—and so can yours.*

Some may say, *"Yeah, I might think about asking Jesus into my life, but I don't have time to spend with God or go to church. I definitely don't have time to read the Bible."* I would argue otherwise. You're reading the last chapter of this book because you made the time. That's proof that you're capable of making time to read. Making time for God is good. I made the time to have Him help me put this memoir down on paper—and believe me, He helped. My story completely pales in comparison to the stories of the Bible, "For everything that was written in the past was written to teach us, so that through the endurance taught in the Scriptures and the encouragement they provide we might have hope."[10]

Read His Word and discover how He restores broken lives. Focus on Him and never underestimate what He can do, or how much He loves us. He's promised to be our constant serenity, peace, and hope. "...we who have fled to Him for refuge can have great confidence as we hold onto the hope that lies before us. This hope is a strong and trustworthy anchor for our souls. It leads us through the curtain into God's inner sanctuary."[11]

Hope means not giving up, but rather reaching out to God. Hope in God promises that you're not alone. Hope in Him introduces us to the promise of eternal life. Hope is strong and makes life beautiful. Hope is the encouragement to press on. I found it, and my steadfast prayer for you is that you'll find it too. I was once told, "Sister, you have a story to share!" It's God's miraculous story, not mine.

To lovers of the truth, nothing can be put before God and Hope in Him.

— Saint Basil

"...but those who hope in the Lord will renew their strength. They will soar on wings like eagles; they will run and not grow weary, they will walk, and not be faint."[14] Read the title of this book, *Halo Found Hope*, and write it down. But before you do, replace "Halo" with *your* name. Put the message in a place where you will see it every day.

Jesus said, "I have told you these things, so that in Me you may have peace. In this world you will have trouble. But take heart! I have overcome the world."[12]

And that's how this Halo found Hope.

Afterward

History, despite its wrenching pain, cannot be unlived, but if faced with courage, need not be lived again.

— Maya Angelou —

I admit that putting this story down on paper wasn't easy. Working with a brain that has a new normal is hard. Trying to write with constant daily interruption as a wife, mom, daughter, sister, and friend made it difficult to stay focused. But every time I started, I asked God to make it His. And He did.

The first six chapters were the most emotionally draining for me to write. In *Called to a Halt*, I had to rehearse and revisit what it was like to learn that I had something in my brain that wasn't supposed to be there. In *Pummeled by Fear*, I grasped onto the stark reality that I might leave those I love—way too soon. Having my life threatened like that was no fun.

In order to write *Into the Hands of God*, I took on the painstaking task of reading through a stack full of details of my surgical encounter. I chose to see what it was like to cut open my skull—to open my brain and take the hidden monster out. It was a story printed with black ink on white paper, but for me, *"This is my head we are talking about!"* Some days I could handle it—other times it shocked me so much that I sobbed. But the silver lining is that I learned firsthand who I am to give thanks to, and I now transparently cherish the One who created us. "I will praise You, for I am fearfully and wonderfully made; Marvelous are Your works, and that my soul knows very well."[1] Reminded of how intricate our bodies are, I completely understand that only God could have made us. And I am so thankful that He cared enough to take the time to do it right.

To put down on paper *The Longest Six Days Ever*, the quest of learning more about my surgery and the lengthy recovery afterward, continued.

I had the honor and privilege of sitting together with my husband across from Dr. Raisis for hours of interview time and a spot of tea. I got to learn what my doctor was "most afraid" of when he took my life into his hands. *He really didn't like where my tumor was located.* While sitting there listening to my husband and Dr. Raisis talk serious, then smile, and laugh, I reflected and removed myself from the conversation for a few moments.

"*I'm alive. I can see, think, talk, and laugh. I get to sit here with my beloved husband across from the skilled surgeon who operated on my brain. This conversation is so different from the one the three of us had the day before the main surgery. Back then we rehearsed the seriousness of potential complications—including death. I remember shaking. I'm not shaking now. Helo, you have so much to be thankful for. Thank you, God.*" Then I rejoined the conversation—I was on the other side of something awful.

In *The Quest for Rehabilitation*, although I was through the surgery, I wasn't finished with the journey. A new normal was yet to be discovered: How to walk, talk, eat, and think again. Now I *love* to skip, laugh, feast, contemplate, and praise, too. Learning how to do so much over again taught me something that I will never forget, and something I can't wait to share with others.

God loves each and every one of us.

Sometimes, it's not until we get to the other side, that we see how much we needed and need God. That is when we realize that He never left and will never leave us after all.

In *Changes, Changes and More Changes* I got to see both sides of a new normal. Physically, I was different—spiritually, I was brand new yet again. But healing does not always take us right back to where we were before the affliction. However, when we let God carry us through adversity we get to see Him with unmatched clarity and we get to know Him. That is beautiful.

In *God is Amazing* through *Hope Found,* I still find myself amazed, each time I read it, at how much God has done in my life. He has changed my perspective. He has amazed me with how much He loves me, how intensely my family loves me and what matters most. Life-changing is too simple to describe this story and what God is capable of doing for all of us. No obstacle is too large, no affliction too grave, to separate us from the love God has for us. Life here is simply a dress rehearsal, but when we allow alterations to be directed by God, the new us discovered, is incredible.

Hope found in God is the only place where searching for it stops.

— Helo

Understated Thank-Yous

Dear God — All accolades go to You. I love You in ways that are sometimes inexplicable because your perfect love draws me to a place of speechless awe. Thank you for being an amazing Heavenly Father and for loving me with patience and faithfulness. Thank you for hearing every prayer I whisper, and for catching every single tear I cry. Thank you for reminding me to keep my focus upon your promises. You know how to remove doubt, replace it with trust, and how to make me strong when I feel like giving up. Thank you for going before me in battle, for never letting me go, and staying close to those I love. Thank you for miraculously keeping me alive and for blessing me with more time to cherish those around me. I am humbled, moved, and shaken. I will try my best to take nothing for granted again. Thank you for your promise that through Jesus, I will never be alone, and will one day enter your eternal Kingdom, a place free from suffering or affliction. There, we will all find everlasting peace, eternal joy, and infinite love. I look forward to dancing in Heaven with your Son, Jesus. When I reflect upon what You have pulled me through, I am brought to tears of joy every time. I know without a single doubt that all hope is found in You.

I love You, God. — *Helo*

Rich, my husband: You are my best friend, the love of my life, an amazing father to our children, and a man moved only by God. In the middle of chaos, you consistently remain calm and encouraging. You find hope in God, and that is contagious. Words will never be enough to thank you for staying by my side and loving me the way that you do. I will always adore, admire, need, and love you.

My cherished children, Lauren, Jordan, and Austin: God blessed me with the gift of raising you three. I am honored to be called your mom. My tenacity to press on came from an incredible longing to return home to you and dad. Thank you for loving me through the ups and downs. I will never go a day without praying for you and telling you how much I love you.

Dad and Mom: I'm honored to have you as my parents. Thank you so much for your dedication and sacrifice as you stood by my side daily. Your love is incredible, and I hope to continue to share the sort of compassion with others that you both know how to give.

Grandma Karin: Thank you for your continual prayers and the support you give to your son, grandchildren, and me. You are a gentle, wise, and caring mother-in-law, and I am so blessed to have you in my life.

My brother, Henk: I love you for your humble, driven walk with Christ. You are a great inspiration to me. Thank you for being by my side.

My sister-in-law, Kristen: Thank you for being a prayer warrior for me when I couldn't be one for myself. I so cherish your prayers and friendship.

Tim and Diane: Thank you for your friendship of a lifetime, heart-to-heart conversations, continual encouragement, and generosity.

All of my extended family and friends: Thank you for your unending willingness to lend a helping hand and prayer. I love you.

Dr. James Raisis: "I am in here." Thank you for being such an incredible instrument in saving my life as my neurosurgeon. You are my earthly hero. Thank you for your exemplary knowledge, wisdom, objectivity, skilled hands, and compassion.

Dr. Calvin Knapp: Thank you for your phenomenal care over the years and for the compassionate way you handled the day of diagnosis. I will never forget it.

Dr. David Tempest: Thank you for directing my rehabilitative quest to learn how to do so much over again.

To the nurses in the Swedish Medical Center ICU and Rehabilitation Unit and Tara, my ENT's nurse: Your heartfelt compassion and relentless care had an enormous effect upon me. "Thank you" does not say enough.

To the countless new acquaintances with whom I have shared my story while in the middle of writing this book: Thank you for your encouragement and motivation to continue.

Mary Grace: Thank you for your generous and compassionate gift of an author shoot. I am stunned by your exceptional, talented approach. I will always remember the comfortable way in which you captured from my heart, a simple reflection of hope. See website at www.marygracelong.com.

A second thank you to my daughter Lauren—my in-house editor: Thank you for editing the very first draft, and drafts that followed. Thanks for your generosity and patience! Your help with this project continues to mean more to me than you will ever know.

Deborah Pless: Thank you for keeping me upbeat while you helped me put clarifying touches on the most difficult content of the manuscript. You made me laugh.

Brenda White: Thank you for continually helping me to place this story before the Lord in prayer—reminding us both that "It is His." Thank you for walking with me as we put beautiful, solid, and final polishing touches on the entire manuscript. I love you for your compassion, wisdom, faith, and life-long friendship.

Chip Kidd: Thank you for making this story strong and simple on the outside, capturing the curious reader to discover the intricacy on the inside. You are one talented book cover designer—it was delightful to work with you.

Notes

Introduction
1.   Music and Lyrics written by Jerry Herman in 1964.
2.   Genesis 1:3
3.   Isaiah 40:31

Chapter One: Brought to a Halt
1.   Psalm 46:10

Chapter Two: Pummeled by Fear
1.   Psalm 91:2, KJV
2.   Isaiah 41:10
3.   Psalm 46:10
4.   Joshua 1:9
5.   G.K. Chesterton
6.   Deuteronomy 31:8, ESV

Chapter Three: Into the Hands of God
1.   Psalm 46:1
2.   John 14:27

Chapter Four: The Longest Six Days Ever
1.   United States Secretary of State 1949-1953
2.   Psalm 30:5

Chapter Six: Changes, Changes and More Changes
1.   American author and civil rights activist (1924-1987)

Chapter Seven: God Is Amazing

1. Psalm 116:8–9, paraphrased
2. Jeremiah 33:6 KJV paraphrased
3. The Complete Tales of Winnie-the-Pooh by A. A. Milne
4. Psalm 119:50 ESV

Chapter Eight: Resilience

1. Psalm 41:3 NKJV
2. Hebrews 4:16, NASB
3. This person's name has been changed for confidentiality.

Chapter Nine: Transparent Disability

1. Hebrews 11:1 NASB
2. This person's name has been changed for confidentiality.

Chapter Ten: He Answers Prayer

1. 1 Chronicles 16:34
2. Jeremiah 33:3
3. Matthew 6:34, paraphrased
4. Psalm 107:28–30, NASB
5. Matthew 6:34
6. Psalm 116:1–2
7. 1 Thessalonians 5:17, KJV
8. Hebrews 12:1-2 NASB

Chapter Eleven: No Complaining

1. 1 Thessalonians 5:18, KJV
2. Philippians 4:8, ESV
3. Psalms 19:14 KJV
4. Ephesians 4:29

5.   Psalm 118:24 NASB

6.   Psalm 32:7

Chapter Twelve: Rich in Love

1.   Luke 23:34

Chapter Thirteen: Seven Blessings

1.   Max Lucado – You are Special

2.   An Orphan's Tale

3.   Jeremiah 29:11

4.   Joshua 1:9 ESV paraphrased

5.   Psalm 18:28 ESV paraphrased

Chapter Fourteen: Avalanche of Post-it® Notes

1.   Isaiah 45:2, KJV paraphrased

2.   Philippians 4:13, KJV paraphrased

Chapter Fifteen: A Parent's Suffering

1.   A Child Dies, Arnold and Gemma 1994, iv, 9, 39

2.   John 3:16, NASB

Chapter Sixteen: Puzzles

1.   1 Peter 5:6 ESV

2.   1 Peter 5:10 ESV

3.   Parkinson Wellness Recovery out of Tucson, AZ founded by Becky Farley PhD and Business Partner Sally Michaels, PT. For more information see pwr4life.org

4.   James 4:14 NASB

5.   Isaiah 53:5

Chapter Seventeen: Intentions

    1.   James 1:12

Chapter Eighteen: Dance with Me, Jesus

    1.   John 14:27

    2.   This person's name has been changed for confidentiality.

    3.   Psalm 103:2–4 NKJV

    4.   Philippians 4:6–7 NKJV

    5.   Psalm 46:10

Chapter Nineteen: Not by Accident

    1.   Psalm 116:8–9

Chapter Twenty: More Than a Survivor

    1.   2 Corinthians 4:8 ESV

    2.   Philippians 4:13 NKJV

    3.   Psalm 28:7, NKJV

    4.   Romans 8:38–39

    5.   Psalm 41:1, NKJV

Chapter Twenty-One: Hope Found

    1.   1 Peter 1:6–7

    2.   Job 11:18, NASB

    3.   2 Corinthians 4:16–17 NASB

    4.   Matthew 6:26

    5.   John 8:32

    6.   Tune added in 1862 by William Bradbury

    7.   1 Peter 5:10

    8.   James 1:2-4 NASB

    9.   1 John 4:8, paraphrased

10. Romans 15:4

11. Hebrews 6:18–19, NLT

12. Isaiah 40:31

13. John 16:33

Afterward

1. Psalm 139:14 NKJV

About the Author

Helo Matzelle is happily married and a devoted mother of three children. She graduated with a Bachelor's Degree from the University of Washington in 1986. She is a dedicated advocate of the National Brain Tumor Society. Helo remains passionate about inspiring others to seek the One in whom true hope is always found. Helo and her family live in Redmond, Washington.

CPSIA information can be obtained
at www.ICGtesting.com
Printed in the USA
FSOW02n1804120315
5694FS